Food for Arthritics

Food for Arthritics
based on Dr Dong's Diet

Judy and Jim Andrews

First published in 1982
by Faber and Faber Limited
3 Queen Square London WC1N 3AU
Printed in Great Britain by
Redwood Burn Ltd Trowbridge Wiltshire
All rights reserved

© Judy and Jim Andrews, 1982

CONDITIONS OF SALE

This book is sold subject to the condition that it shall not, by way of trade or otherwise, be lent, resold, hired out or otherwise circulated without the publisher's prior consent in any form of binding or cover other than that in which it is published and without a similar condition including this condition being imposed on the subsequent purchaser

British Library Cataloguing in Publication Data

Andrews, Judy
  Food for Arthritics: based on Dr Dong's Diet
  1. Arthritis – Diet therapy – Recipes
  I. Title II. Andrews, Jim
  616.7'220654.   RC.933
  ISBN 0–571–11876–3
  ISBN 0–571–11911–5 Pbk

With sincere gratitude to
DR COLLIN H. DONG
without whose genius
our life would be in ruins

Contents

PART 1

INTRODUCTION *by Jim Andrews*	11
Dr Dong's Diet	26
Eating Out	32
Entertaining at Home	34
Travelling	35
Tips on 'Cheating'	36
PUTTING THE DIET INTO PRACTICE *by Judy Andrews*	39
Finding the Right Food	39

PART 2: RECIPE SECTION

USING THE RECIPES	51
Adapting Ordinary Recipes	51
General Notes on the Recipes	52
DRINKS, HOT AND COLD	54
BREAKFAST DISHES	57
BAKING BREADS AND SCONES	60
SPREADS	64
FIRST COURSE DISHES	66
SOUPS	71
MAIN COURSE FISH DISHES	79

CONTENTS

MAIN COURSE SHELLFISH DISHES	93
MAIN COURSES WITHOUT FISH	100
VEGETABLE DISHES	116
SALAD DISHES	152
SAUCES	157
PUDDINGS AND SWEETS	160
PASTRY, CAKES, BUNS AND BISCUITS	166
USEFUL BOOKS	181
INDEX	183
DR DONG'S DIET	188

PART ONE

Introduction

by Jim Andrews

People who suffer from arthritic joints know only too well what it is to live from day to day with the particular brand of aching agony that this awful yet little-understood ailment inflicts. Even so, with some twenty-odd forms of the disease to study, medical science has found difficulty both in isolating the causes and in finding a truly curative treatment. Some things help, such as ordinary soluble aspirin and stronger drugs like cortisone, but they can have distressing side-effects, excellent though they undoubtedly are.

So how would it be if, instead of taking medicines of any kind, arthritic people could eliminate the pain, misery and stiffnesses, and return to an active, happy life just by eating—or rather, by not eating—certain ordinary foodstuffs?

I agree that such an idea at first sounds highly unlikely, but read on; there is no 'quack' remedy involved, just a completely normal process of the human body. As I sit comfortably typing this page with totally pain-free fingers and spine, my relaxed elbows sharing movement after movement with equally mobile wrists, I know from firsthand experience how simply this apparent miracle really can be achieved.

Let me tell you a little about myself. As a teenage schoolboy I was fond of physical training, and developed quite powerful muscles on my stocky, 5ft 9in frame. Speed of action was learnt through a liking for playing squash. Having been brought up by the sea, a passion for sailing led in time to my becoming a successful enough racing skipper.

INTRODUCTION

In 1961 I met a girl who was every bit as keen, and so good a helmswoman that I was careful never to race against her. We got married in 1962, and took to cruising.

By 1974 I was aged forty, and, with Judy and our three daughters, was living in an ancient fishing village tucked away up a superbly beautiful sea-loch on the west coast of Scotland. Our modest cruising boat was moored close by, unless we were out there, thrilling to the thrust of the slanting sails as she soared and swooped over the waves, taking us among the heather-scented isles, or across the Firths and Sounds to the boisterous Sea of the Hebrides. Normally I did all the heavy work on board, such as heaving up the anchor or struggling with wildly flogging canvas on wet and lurching decks, to change sails when a rising wind became too strong for my family to manage. And we had exciting plans in mind for more extended cruises, southwards to the sun.... Daydreams maybe, but viable ones—then.

As an author and sailing journalist, whatever time I spent afloat was seldom wasted, for inevitably I was able to turn some of the experiences thus gained into magazine articles or technical books, and even the occasional novel. Often woven into the last was the knowledge won from the other hobby Judy and I so contentedly shared, which was archaeology. This too could demand exertions: kneeling for hours with bent back, delicately excavating with a trowel some treasured fragment from the bottom of a damp cutting, or perhaps trekking on foot for miles over the wild hills to inspect or seek out some strange Bronze Age or Neolithic burial site. Though both rather heavier than we should have been, because Judy enjoys cooking, we were pretty fit. Or was I?

It was in coming down hills that I began to encounter the first signs of joint trouble. A sharp, piercing pain would unexpectedly lance through a knee, making me gasp aloud, stumble, and stop in my tracks. On board the boat too, while kneeling to some job with the engine, I had once or twice felt

INTRODUCTION

a wickedly sudden prick at the base of a kneecap, rather as though I had inadvertently knelt on a drawing-pin.

Soon there were other effects, which for me were still more unnerving. My fingers, so fond of playing musical instruments and of typing to supplement our income, grew gradually painful in their end joints, so that even the affectionate hold of a gentle young daughter was enough to make me stifle an involuntary yell. Typing became increasingly difficult.

I didn't know what was the matter, and neither did my doctor, for at that stage even X-rays failed to show up anything unusual. With one aunt severely crippled by arthritis, and a mother whose spine had all but solidified before her early death, I had my suspicions; but comfortingly there was no medical proof whatever to as much as suggest that this was happening to me.

As writing had become such a problem, in order to boost family funds and have more time sailing, Judy and I set up our own small yacht-charter business, hiring out our little ship to groups of happy people for whom I went along as skipper, cook, navigator, steward, and shore guide, and for a time it all went superbly. Except that even when lying in my bunk at night, and in my bed at home between charters, I began to experience severe aches in my ribs and between my shoulder-blades. With more and more loss of sleep, the job of coping with what was now almost continuous discomfort in fingers, wrists, knees, and finally elbows, while remaining able to chat cheerily with our guests, became all but impossible.

At last I could barely manage the sailing; going down the few steps into the cabin or climbing up on deck to shorten sail were acutely painful activities for which I had to steel myself minutes in advance of making the attempt. I no longer felt I could be sure of coping in a gale, when even in normal weather, every movement of the boat came like a sledge-hammer blow on my upper spine.

The most frightening thing of all was the sheer speed with

INTRODUCTION

which I was becoming progressively more disabled. We had no idea at this stage that the diet on board of largely tinned and processed 'convenience' food was actively accelerating the trouble.

To my utter dismay, even our own family cruise in the summer of 1978, when I could hardly have had a more able crew, proved a disaster. The continual, exhausting pain made me short-tempered and restless. Cruising no longer made sense. In despair, we sold our beloved ship—and all my daydreams with her. . . .

By September of that year I was having to be helped out of a chair, into my socks, up the stairs, down the path from our high-perched house, and in and out of baths, in the hot water of which I seemed to gain some degree of blissful release. But at only forty-five this was quite ridiculous! Again I went to my doctor, complaining of the chest-pains which woke me each time I rolled on my side in my sleep (he knew about the other things), and once more I did the rounds of blood-tests and radiography.

A week went by, and he called me to the surgery. Swivelling on my stick (my dear stick, without which I was now all but immobilized), I managed to sit down, and he held up the X-ray of my spine, tapping at the grey ghosts of its upper vertebrae with a finger. Then he looked sideways at me.

'Needn't beat about the bush,' he said softly. 'Arthritis. There, there, and here as well. The blood samples were OK, so it's not rheumatoid, which is something; but I'm afraid it's pretty generalized.' He sat down and looked me straight in the eyes. 'There isn't a lot we can do to help you, Jim,' he added bluntly.

'There's nothing . . .?' I began, clutching wildly for aid.

He shook his head. 'Some day, maybe. There's a lot of research going on.' He took a deep breath. 'Aspirin is really the best thing for you just now, though not more than eighteen a day, and no more than four at a time. And I can prescribe a muscle-relaxant which may ease things a bit. Eventually you will have to go on to cortisone—it's the only

INTRODUCTION 15

answer we have at the moment—but that's some way off yet. You don't want to start until you really have to.'

'Thank you for being straight with me,' I replied.

He studied my face for a few seconds longer. 'Good luck,' he said solemnly.

I left the surgery in a rapidly developing state of shock, which of course did nothing at all to improve things. I had inwardly known the truth myself for weeks, but having it so concisely confirmed was devastating. It suddenly sank right in that, short of some kind of miracle, I was condemned to live the full-time hell of arthritic pain for the rest of my days. It was an almost unthinkable prospect. In only four short years, from being a healthy, active sailorman, bursting with the joys of being part of an enchanting, intriguing world of wildlife and wind, mountain and sea, I had suddenly turned into a crotchety old man, puffing and blowing with every move, and annoying myself and everyone around me.

The doctor's kind wish for luck, even if it was almost all he could do to help, must indeed have been deeply sincere, for in only a matter of a few days fortune rose like the sun in the shape of Judy waving a copy of *Here's Health* magazine, which she had picked up in a health food shop.

'Jim,' she began, a trifle hesitantly, 'you'll probably think this is the crankiest idea yet, but there's an article here by a woman who has been on some weird diet, and found her arthritis has practically cleared up. I don't suppose you'd try it, but...' Judy, if anyone did, knew very well how hopeless I was at sticking to the like of slimming diets, and also how disappointed I had been at the various recent attempts of one or two 'fringe medicine' people to assist me with the arthritis problem.

I glanced up from my chair. 'Look,' I said. 'I don't care how "quack" or odd it sounds, I'll try anything now if it's going to work. Is there any way you think it could harm me? Has it got all the right vitamins and things?' She comes from a medical family, and has always been keenly interested in nutrition, as the good health of our offpsring bears witness. 'What does it consist of, anyway?'

'No meat,' she said, reading from a list of 'Dos and Don'ts'. 'No dairy produce, nor any sort of animal food, even milk. No fruit and no . . .'

'No *fruit*?' I exclaimed, astonished.

'No chocolate either,' she went on, 'and no chemical additives—which just could be the hardest bit to cope with, nowadays.'

My mind raced ahead. No more pork pies. No more apples, bananas, pears, or . . . 'What about vitamin C? What *can* I eat, for goodness sake?'

'Plenty of fresh vegetables, raw if possible, and all kinds of fish, even shellfish. There's ample protein in that.'

'Judy . . .' I began, and hesitated. Since infancy, my two most unfavourite kinds of food were fish and vegetables. I turned to gaze through the window over the loch that I loved—and at once it was as though someone had struck me between the shoulder-blades with a blunt axe. Straightening with a sharp intake of breath, I paused, rigid with pain. An icy sweat prickled over my scalp. 'Let's try it,' I gasped. 'It just might do something, though for the life of me I can't see how. Let's have a look at that article.'

Relaxing somewhat, I read how Mary Laver had been taken over by rheumatoid arthritis until she was in a far worse condition than even I was in, and had then come across Dr Dong's Diet. Even so, I completely failed to believe that just by selective eating, the appalling effects of the disease could be as easily and rapidly overcome as she described. Yet here was a picture of her, energetically playing badminton, apparently taken only a month or two after she had started the diet.

I was distracted by the muffled sound of flogging canvas from beyond the window, followed by the ring and clatter of sheet-winches, as a yacht tacked close inshore below the house, and her crew vigorously re-trimmed the sails. No more chocolate or puddings, I thought. Maybe not even

INTRODUCTION

wine, as that was fruit-based (and being half French, I had been brought up from childhood to enjoy good wine with a meal now and then). And only fish and veg. . . . Yet, as I watched the yacht lean, and go loping away over a surging bow-wave, heading out across the blue water towards a certain delightful island anchorage near the far shore, something within me gave a firm nudge, sparking just a tiny glimmer of hope.

'You don't *have* to try it,' said Judy.

'I will, if you can cook it for me. For a fortnight, anyway. According to this, that ought to be long enough to tell me if it'll make any difference at all, though I honestly can't see how it might.'

That was the beginning and, as I write, it was about two years ago. Last weekend, Judy and I took our lively, twelve-foot sailing dinghy for a lengthy exploration of the Urr estuary, on the Solway Firth. There was a brisk breeze blowing and the little craft was quite a handful in the gusts, necessitating quick actions and rapid dodging under the boom as we short-tacked among the winding channels. But then, Judy and I are remarkably fit, despite being (very) middle-aged.

It had taken only five days from starting the diet for Judy to notice what I had already begun to feel.

'You're moving more easily' she said, and it was true. And a fortnight later, after sticking faithfully to every recommendation of Dr Dong's Diet and Mary Laver's article, I only required my stick if going for a walk. I thought it was time I could maybe cheat a little, for I longed to bite into a crisp, juicy apple. I did, and within half an hour I was again in dire trouble with my back. Finger joints began stinging with pain; knees went weak with aching, and muscles in all limbs were tightening up. I was back to 'square one', and it took another three days to regain something like the freedom I had previously won, following the diet implicitly once more.

A few weeks later, during a discussion about what it might

be in various foods that seemed to cause me difficulty, we found ourselves wondering if in the case of meat it could simply be the animal fat which was harmful. Judy remarked that we still had a venison fillet in the freezer—the prime piece and all that remained of a roe-deer which a forester friend had most generously given us the previous year. Venison is just about the least fatty of all four-legged animal meats, and when uncooked all the fat can clearly be seen in thin white streaks. With great care, Judy removed every trace of these, and the resulting dish was utter perfection in flavour and texture as far as I was concerned; an evening meal to remember. But in more ways than one. Inside a couple of hours, I had to be helped upstairs to bed, in the most dreadful pain.

After I had recovered, in a few days' time, further discussion revealed uncertainty on both our parts as to whether the awful effects of these (delicious) experiments had perhaps been a psychological reaction, rather than a true one, particularly as the pain had returned so very quickly, albeit surprisingly, but we soon found there was nothing imaginary about it. As the days went on, inevitably I accidentally consumed the occasional 'wrong' thing—tinned goods containing an acid preservative or some obscure chemical additive, or perhaps some processed fish laced with monosodium glutamate—and the last substance always produced the most violent and excruciating reaction of all. Or else we ate out, and the cook used pepper. On more than one occasion I found myself fighting not to wince as I struggled to rise from the dining table—once in our own home after eating a little tinned, but extremely delectable, smoked salmon, which as a seafood treat had been specially brought to me by a visiting member of the family.

But we persevered, simply because as long as we stuck to it properly, the result was so incredible and so rewarding. (I say 'we', because by now Judy had 'gone on the diet' herself when there were just the two of us at home, purely for convenience.) And gradually, as we learnt how to prepare a

INTRODUCTION 19

greater variety of dishes, we ate more and more deliciously.

Despite lack of success with 'slimming diets' in the past, both of us gently but steadily lost excess fat, and became lighter, for that is one of the added and very important bonuses of this kind of food; but there are more intriguing effects still. Very soon we each began to feel noticeably far more mentally alert than ever before, and I regained an almost forgotten degree of stamina which I had last known as a teenager.

There were other curiosities. Judy's persistent catarrh cleared up, though it always returned during school holidays when the girls were at home—until she traced it to taking the milk and other dairy products which were then in the house. And a troublesome condition in both her wrists has also ceased to occur, unless she is tempted by the girls' bowl of citrus fruits. So the diet is unquestionably good for both of us! For Judy, however, the greatest benefit must certainly be in not having to act virtually as nursemaid to a helpless, bad-tempered husband, for, to my continued astonishment, and just like Mary Laver, I am at least as active as I was before the arthritis started to take hold of me.

I move almost completely painlessly again; I walk the hills and forests; go archaeologizing; sail with all the old verve and enthusiasm I had before, often single-handed; and no longer need people to heave me up or help me down. To be totally honest, although with care I am able to lift heavy things, there are some jobs, such as those tough ones involving contortions on the leaping, bouncing, slippery deck of a yacht at sea, which I am still unwilling to tackle.

At home, however, I can once more mow grass, do the weeding, paint the house (what a job that was!), and play keyboard and stringed instruments with all my old blissful lack of skill. My elbows flex; knees function normally (if a trifle noisily at times), except on really steep inclines or steps; and my spine, though none too flexible due to having fused vertebrae for part of its length, causes only occasional dis-

INTRODUCTION

comfort, usually because I have eaten some minute quantity of something I shouldn't.

This happened just the other day. Pain developed suddenly in knee and elbow joints—yet we were both sure I had eaten nothing I hadn't been in the recent habit of enjoying safely. Then I recalled how especially tasty a new packet of sesame biscuits we had sampled that morning had been. Suspicions aroused, we hunted out the wrapper, and read again the once familiar list of ingredients. The manufacturers had seen fit to 'improve' them with the new addition of cocoa-butter. And there, of course, was the answer.

It is at times like that, that I am forcibly reminded of something one must understand from the start. *Good though it is, the diet is not a cure.* All it does—and for me, and countless other people, is doing—is to let one live again like any normal, reasonably fit, vivacious person. The joy of that is wonderful.

Ah, you might well ask, but isn't it *awfully* difficult, living with such a complicated diet?

Well, of course there are problems. Eating out is one and, by extension, travelling can be another. Buying the right sort of food is a constant challenge, always making sure that the content is 'safe'. One becomes an inveterate label-reader. But I have long since stopped drooling over shelves of my once most favourite delicacies; I know only too well how quickly my body would be wracked with agony if I ever tried them again. The very thought appals!

As Judy said, it is not a question of *having* to be on this diet, in the sense of anyone making me. I just *want* to continue with it, because whether the medical profession as a whole does or doesn't understand why or how it works, I know that for me and lots of other arthritic folk, it *does*. I still have the arthritis, there is no mistake about that, but I look as normal as ever I did, walk quickly, stepping out freely, and do more or less whatever I want in the way of exercise, be it swimming, dinghy-racing or even a little occasional real sea-going, as crew in friends' boats.

INTRODUCTION

If you are still reading, I imagine it is because you either care for, or are, someone who suffers from a form of arthritis, and because you now can't wait to know more about the diet itself, and its source.

Collin H. Dong, MD, was born of an American mother and a Chinese father. A fully qualified physician, by the age of only thirty-five he had become entirely crippled by multiple forms of arthritis. He was confined to a wheelchair, grossly distorted, and in constant torment both as the result of pain, and the effects of a terrible, associated skin condition. After developing the diet, he regained extreme fitness, and at the age of over seventy habitually played a quick round of golf each morning, before dashing off to deal with his busy surgery.

In the midst of his earlier distress, however, when all available 'treatments' and medicines had failed to bring any relief or improvement, he had suddenly recalled an old Chinese saying of his father's, which, roughly translated, read: 'Sickness comes in through the mouth, and catastrophe comes out of the mouth.' One may smile at the last part, but the first is the bit that really caught Collin Dong's attention, so that he began gradually eliminating from his daily food intake all those things which the Chinese doctors of old had always considered could produce allergic reactions. Such as animal products, for a start; then fruit. His condition improved, to the astonishment of all those trying to care for him, and by trial and (most painful) error, he ended up with the diet that today bears his name, and keeps literally thousands of once severely handicapped arthritic patients fit, active and virtually completely free of the pain that had once wrecked their lives. And I suppose that every one of them started out on the diet as sceptical as both Judy and I were, and indeed as most present-day medical people still tend to be, despite the fact that doctors in general are taking more and more interest in what their patients are eating nowadays.

INTRODUCTION

The point is that this is a properly balanced diet—worked out by a qualified and highly successful medical practitioner—rather than a vague idea put about by some 'health nut'. And as it involves no medicines of any kind, even the most reserved of conventional British doctors will admit 'at least it can do you no harm', usually adding, 'if you even *believe* it's doing you good, then it probably will'.

For myself, I don't know or particularly care whether there may be an element of psychology in it, or not. All I can say is that at first I certainly did *not* believe what I read in Mary Laver's article (and she will forgive me for saying so, since she knows how grateful I am to her for writing it). I was indeed only a little more inclined to be convinced when we obtained and read the two books she mentioned, namely *New Hope for the Arthritic*, and *The Arthritic's Cookbook*, both by Collin H. Dong and June Banks, and published in the United Kingdom by Granada. Actually trying the diet, and getting the astounding results I did, was for me the real and quite undeniable 'proof of the pudding'.

All one can say in layman's terms is that the sort of food normally eaten by Europeans contains a number of more or less toxic substances, as well as many known allergens. Most people's digestive systems are able to cope with these without problems, at least in youth and middle age, but for reasons not yet understood, a large number cannot. Today there are many sad cases of even very young children suffering from arthritis, and where elderly people are concerned, one almost *expects* them to become arthritic, to a greater or, one hopes, lesser extent.

Most of us know of at least one person who is allergic, say, to pollen in the air they breathe or, where food is concerned, to eggs or cows' milk.

In compiling his diet, Dr Dong has simply eliminated these and other less obvious items, so that the body has every possible chance of using its own natural recuperative powers to the full, to sort out the disorders so caused.

Before anyone starts out to follow this diet, I feel I must

INTRODUCTION

stress most earnestly that *it could be highly dangerous suddenly to stop using medicines which have been prescribed*—particularly where cortisone or any related steroid-type of drug is concerned—and to try and rely immediately on the diet alone. Many of these modern drugs are likely to produce very severe problems indeed if the supply is interrupted in any way. It is therefore absolutely *vital* that if you are under this kind of treatment, *you should keep on taking the recommended doses, for at least the first fortnight of going on the diet.*

After that, if your condition is showing definite signs of improving you could approach your physician and ask for the dosage to be gradually reduced as he/she thinks fit, in view of your improvement. Eventually the time will come when it is *safe* for you to stop taking whatever it is altogether—but it would be madness to make even the slightest drug-intake reduction without full medical approval. It is *extremely important* to understand this.

Just in case you have been wondering, I do occasionally take a couple of aspirin, perhaps once every couple of months or so, and usually because I have eaten something that I shouldn't. In fact I used to take aspirin far more frequently, to combat migraine attacks—which have quite deserted me now.

There are initial side-effects that may occur in some people when the diet is first fully adhered to. Judy and I both noticed that after a few weeks, the skin on the backs of our hands commenced to take on a rather papery look, but this was only due to our losing fat—presumably from our hands as well as the more obvious places—and has since cleared up. In fact, we *think* our skins look healthier than ever before.

We also found, but for a while only, that if we got scratched or cut, for instance when gardening, we had a tendency to bleed slightly more than we might previously have expected—so this is something which people who bleed easily should watch carefully. Again, the condition was only temporary.

24 INTRODUCTION

Because we then lived in a fairly remote part of the west of Scotland, where it was extremely difficult to get vegetables of any variety or freshness, salads in particular being hard to obtain, we ran a little short of vitamin C, and had to take supplementary tablets. These, of course, contain ascorbic acid, which is not ideal in concentrated form. For business reasons we have since moved to the Solway area, where all sorts of fresh greens are normally plentiful and I can eat raw vegetables every day, so that my intake of natural vitamin C is now adequate.

Though it did not happen to either of us, we know of some arthritic people who, shortly after starting on the diet, complained of a foul taste in their mouths. This too soon passes.

One can hardly expect to alter one's eating habits so radically without some temporary loss of condition. Any farmer will tell you that if he has, for instance, to change a pig's diet (no matter how much for the better in the long run), initially the animal's general condition will very slightly drop, before picking up and improving as its digestive system becomes, so to speak, acclimatized. It is just the same with humans (who are surprisingly similar inside!).

The thing is, the sooner you go completely on to the diet, the sooner the toxic poisons derived from animal fats, fruit acids, and particularly chemical additives, will leave you. Then, and only then, can the often astonishingly vivid improvement begin. And the beauty of it is that the improvement is then one which your body is constructing for itself—completely naturally.

Exercise is vital to fitness, just as the correct diet is, and should be considered as an equally important part of dealing with the problem of arthritis. However, the very word often strikes as much horror into the soul of those unused to exercise as does the word 'diet' to any normal food-lover.

With those seriously afflicted almost any kind of exercise may already have become a thing of the past, and here, as Dr Dong's Diet begins to make moving about more and more easy, there are dangers to be carefully avoided. Getting

INTRODUCTION

around the house is not a bad form of exercise for those who have been very immobilized, but stairs should be attempted with extra caution at first, whether going up or down. Any long-out-of-use muscle is weak in two ways: ability and actual tissue strength. It may be quite easily torn or damaged, so whenever you do start to feel like getting around, take things very gently at first. If walking further than just around the house or garden, do not attempt more than fifty or a hundred yards the first time (if that), and then in a day or two you could try extending it to, say, the same distance twice, once in the morning, and again later in the afternoon. Not more than that. In time, the walk can be lengthened and very, very cautiously speeded up.

The principal trouble with walking is the jolting caused to knees, hips and spine at every step, so wear the spongiest, bounciest footwear you can get hold of to minimize the jarring. I still go for walks with a stout stick, because I found my balance deteriorated in the period of inactivity before I went on to the diet, and because even now, two years later, if I twist a knee awkwardly when crossing rough ground or climbing steps, it can momentarily let me down, and the stick is then my saving grace. By the way, I find it better not to 'swing' the stick, but rather to grip it firmly, and plonk it down in time with the opposite foot's every step. This gives maximum aid and introduces a brisk and steady rhythm to the tread.

As muscle slowly builds and weight comes down, more energetic activities once more become possible, though if the spine has been affected it seems there may always be the need to avoid sudden jolts or twists. Try cycling. A good bike on a smooth road surface is astonishingly exercising to lungs and heart, as well as to muscles and joints, yet provides fewer jerks than does walking. But again, do take it very softly initially. The main thing is to take *some* exercise every day, if at all possible.

Let's see now what the diet *really* means, and how to turn what may at first sight look like a dismaying form of

INTRODUCTION

deprivation into some marvellously varied and extremely tasty dishes.

Note: The list that follows has been slightly adapted for use in the UK. A highly important part of the diet is its weight-reducing ability. Since, therefore, it is better to miss out a few items which might not cause pain directly than to eat even a little of something that could, and because frequent consumption of things like pasta dishes and alcohol tends to put weight on, these are recommended for *occasional* use only. So is the white flesh of birds which, though not fattening, is in our experience best taken only now and then, and in very small quantities.

We are, however, all different, and what any one arthritic individual finds he or she can or cannot get away with will only be determined in time, by careful (and sometimes painful) experiment.

The important thing initially is to follow the 'must not eat' and 'can eat' part of Dr Dong's Diet *implicitly* for the first few weeks, to give your system a chance to adapt and benefit.

DR DONG'S DIET

(Reprinted for quick reference at the end of the book, p. 188)

MUST NOT EAT:
Meat in any form, including broth
Dairy products (milk, cream, butter, cheese, yogurt, whey).*
Egg-yolks
Fruit of any kind, including tomatoes
Chocolate
Dry-roasted nuts (the process involves monosodium glutamate)
Pepper (definitely)
Vinegar, or any other acid

* The lecithin in margarine is acceptable, but whey is not. Beware of this.

INTRODUCTION 27

Most alcoholic beverages
Soft drinks (where they contain additives, fruit products or colouring) Man-made 'chemical' additives (flavourings, preservatives, colourings); this applies above all to *monosodium glutamate*

CAN EAT:

All fish, including shellfish
All vegetables, including avocados
Parsley, onions, garlic, bayleaf, or any other of the herbs
Vegetable oils (especially safflower and corn oils) and pure vegetable fat
Margarine free from milk solids (whey) and forbidden additives
Egg-whites—only
Honey
Sugar (preferably undyed brown), syrup, etc.
Bread and other baked products containing no forbidden additives
Flour of any kind
Rice of all kinds
Soya bean products such as Textured Vegetable Protein (T.V.P.) when free from forbidden additives
Nuts and sunflower seeds
Tea and coffee, taken without milk
Plain soda water
Pure salt (beware of additives in table salt)

CAN OCCASIONALLY EAT:

A little breast of chicken or turkey, and chicken broth
Small amount of wine in cooking
Small drink of whisky, rum, vodka, and possibly white wine (not red)
Very small pinch of spicy seasoning, such as curry powder, mustard, etc.
Pasta such as noodles, spaghetti, macaroni (when present, the amount of egg in these is small)

INTRODUCTION

If you are now left wondering, as we at first glance were, how you would ever get through a day on that lot, here are two sample days' menus, including a dinner-party menu.

DAY ONE

Breakfast
Poached white of egg on toast (p. 58)
Slice of wholemeal bread, spread with vegetable fat or a little olive oil, and honey
Black coffee, or tea

Elevenses
Cup of black coffee
Home-made biscuit

Lunch
Cream of Sweetcorn Soup (p. 76)
Lettuce, grated carrot, cucumber, cress, etc.
Wholemeal bread, 'Vegerine' (p. 64), peanut butter, honey
Water, or home-made ginger-beer

Tea
China tea such as Keemun, or Lapsang Souchong
Rock bun

Supper
Grilled fillets of whiting
Cauliflower in white sauce
'Vichy'-style carrots
Baked potato
Plain meringue
Black coffee or tea

DAY TWO

Breakfast
Bowl of porridge with brown sugar
Toast, 'Vegerine' (p. 64), thin spread of ginger sauce
Black coffee or tea

INTRODUCTION 29

Elevenses
Cup of Postum or similar grain-based beverage
Home-made biscuit

Lunch
Tinned pink salmon
Salad
Water biscuits and honey
Soda water

Tea
Jasmine-blossom tea
Slice of coffee cake

Dinner party
Assorted hors d'oeuvres
Shrimp Flan (p. 94), served with roast potatoes, sprouts, mushrooms
Glass of white wine
Meringue Nests (p. 163)
Black coffee

Not bad, I think you'll agree. And we haven't forgotten those special family occasions. (Who could?) Take Christmas, for example:

CHRISTMAS DINNER

Consommé (p. 71)
Roast Turkey (p. 101)
Chestnut roast (Nut Roast recipe, p. 101–2)
Roast potatoes (done in separate tin, *not* round the turkey)
Brussels sprouts and/or peas
Mince Tarts (p. 164) served with rum-flavoured Trex 'Cream' Filling (p. 170)
Coffee

INTRODUCTION

Breakfasts are never much of a problem, though the variations are somewhat limited. By using a soya plant milk from tins (obtainable from health food shops), one can enjoy the unadulterated commercial breakfast cereals (see p. 42). And one's white of egg can be treated in a number of ways. Since marmalade is 'out' (fruit), one is rather stuck with certain ginger-based products (though go very sparingly with this rather potent substance, for the good of your kidneys), or honey, of which fortunately nowadays there is a wide variety of flavours to choose. As to coffee, there are many kinds. Except for special occasions, we normally prefer decaffeinated brands, which do not over-excite the heart muscles. Indian teas tend to be harsher than China teas when taken without milk; Judy gives our personal preferences on page 54. Take care, though; not all teas are free from added colouring or unspecified flavourings, so *do read the label!*

Our lunches tend mostly to be of a salad or 'bread-and-spread' nature, especially in summer. If a suitable margarine cannot be found (see p. 47) we make up our own 'Vegerine' mix (p. 64) which, though pretty tasteless, has much the same effect in use as a base spread. A thin smear of it, topped with peanut butter, can be made quite delicious by the further addition of a layer of sliced beetroot, cucumber, or even honey. Peanut butter contains a very high level of protein and, with no animal meat or cheese in this diet, protein intake must be very carefully maintained. Besides, one develops a considerable taste for peanut butter applied as above. (I have to admit that I find it impossibly 'tacky' when it is spread on bread on its own, but on top of 'Vegerine' or margarine it is very good.) Potted yeast extracts such as Marmite make excellent spreads, but hunt around in your health food store because there are many different brands available, giving a range of flavours.

We have our main meal in the evening and here feel we can sometimes lash out a bit. Because meat is expensive compared with fish, and one is not buying fruit to eat on its

INTRODUCTION 31

own or for the making of puddings, one can afford occasionally to buy top-quality fish—sea-trout or salmon, rainbow trout, prawns, or even more exotic things—as a treat. And for the same reason, one can maybe go a little mad on special vegetables now and then. A normal evening meal in our family now consists of at least two, but more probably three or even four, different vegetables, as well as the fish or whatever. We eat raw vegetables at least once a day, and feel this is important.

Bread can be a bit of a problem, depending on where you live. Experiment will show, but you may find as I did that even commercially baked wholemeal bread can contain some harmful additives for the arthritic. White commercial loaves in Britain almost always contain 'improvers' such as ascorbic acid, as well as other additives. It may be possible to seek out some small local 'home bakery' which makes its own loaves, and where you can find, or possibly have baked specially, a small batch of wholemeal bread, free of additives, milk and lard, which you can take home and freeze. Baking your own yeast bread is time-consuming, though not at all difficult once you are in the way of it (p. 60–1). We find making soda bread very much quicker, and again have given what we think is a particularly delicious recipe on page 62.

Commercially baked biscuits are another problem. There are hardly any sweet kinds that the arthritic on this diet can safely use, if only because many firms do not supply ingredients lists, either at all or in sufficient detail to let one be *sure* of the contents. All the same, by careful reading, one can find some biscuits suitable for the diet (see p. 44). However, Judy has concocted a number of 'safe' home recipes which I can heartily recommend—in small quantities. The almond, the vanilla and coffee, and the rum and oatmeal are my special favourites. Sound nice, don't they?

Bought cakes, ice-creams and the like are, alas, just not on. They're full of everything the Dong Dieter must not have. Commercially made sweets rank among the 'must nots', but I have found one or two exceptions in peppermint form;

INTRODUCTION

Fox's Glacier Mints and Polo seem (note the word 'seem') to be all right, as do Marks and Spencer's and Nuttall's After Dinner Mints. Just remember that *arthritic people should not eat sweets at all*. It's so terribly bad for the figure *and* for the arthritic joints which have then to bear the extra weight. But well . . . just once in a while, like on one's birthday, it would be a poor thing if there wasn't something one could have by way of luxury.

EATING OUT

The biggest difficulty comes when it is necessary to eat out, away from home. When invited to a friend's house for a meal adherence to the diet can be quite embarrassing. If you just keep quiet, and eat whatever is put before you, the chances are you will be in severe pain before the meal is over, and if you are like me, may even need help to get up when it is time to go. This could be acutely worrying for your host. And if you only pick at your food, and try to eat little bits of oddments you think you can safely select, your hostess will feel hurt.

We believe it better to be totally open the moment the invitation comes, and to explain that there are a great number of things you simply *must not* eat. If the invitation is still pressed, you can then ask if it would be possible for you to have something liked tinned tuna, or grilled fish with salad—without pepper, butter, or any sauce or dressing. (You leave on your plate the tomato, egg-yolk and lemon which usually appears with a fish dish.) Explain that commercially breaded or battered seafood contains monosodium glutamate which you're afraid won't do, in case that is what springs to mind.

If a bird of some kind is on the menu, then of course you can take a very little of the white breast meat (only), with

INTRODUCTION 33

again a little salad without dressing. And you don't eat the sweet (unless they can provide you with plain meringue). It is probably best not to take the soup either, if that has led the meal—unless you are quite sure none of the 'must nots' is in it. On such occasions I usually explain that I eat very little anyway, and that is often accepted. (I have once or twice come home after such an evening out, and made a snack to 'catch up' on a virtually uneaten dinner!)

Hotel and restaurant meals are another matter. Where food is actually prepared on the premises by a good cook or chef, one can ask the waiter if this or that dish could be simplified to exclude the pepper, the tomatoes, the sauce or dressing, etc., and mostly I have found everyone only too happy to help—even if I sometimes still have to lift aside the lettuce contaminated by the inevitable wedge of lemon, and scrape from the skin of my trout an evil sprinkling of black pepper! One may have to forego any kind of 'starter' if there is nothing suitable, and will almost certainly have to miss out on the 'selection of sweets from the trolley', all of which undoubtedly contain either cream, chocolate or fruit. A very good meal can probably still be enjoyed—and without the uncomfortable aftermath of feeling over-fed at the end of it.

It's in those cafés and restaurants where most of the menu comes frozen, or pre-packed and pre-prepared, simply to be brought to temperature in a micro-wave oven before serving, that I find I am so often completely and utterly out of luck. Which is why, when such an outing seems likely, I always have with me a little pot of my 'Vegerine', some water-biscuits or Ryvita, and a small tin of pink salmon, to tide me over. At Chinese restaurants (of which my family is exceedingly fond), most of the food is heavily laced with monosodium glutamate, or some acid-based sauce, so Judy makes in advance a small vacuum-flask of Chinese-Style Fish (p. 84), which I take with me to pour over the plate of boiled or fried rice, explaining first to the waiter, of course, simply out of courtesy, what the problem is. I have never received any sign of objection on their part, and other diners

34 INTRODUCTION

at once assume that I am on some weird diet, and don't mind either.

Where arthritic children are concerned, the problem is a particularly tough one. Alas, all the sweet things and ice-creams and so forth that the very young normally gorge themselves on at party times are 'out'. So are the currently popular savoury sausages, the yogurts, and most soft drinks. However, the arthritic child can still enjoy some kind of party fare. We suggest some savouries on pages 105–7, followed by a variety of cakes and biscuits (pp. 169–79). Soft drinks can be concocted too, using soda water as a base and, for instance, the juice of lemon balm leaves, or homemade ginger-beer (p. 55). Other things can be provided for the non-arthritic guests, especially in the drinks line; but do be careful not to create jealousies which could spoil the day.

Arthritic children living on this diet will quite probably be made by their contemporaries to feel rather cranky, especially since if they are invited to parties they will almost certainly have to take along some of their own food and drink. The best way to get round this (having explained things to the hostess so that she understands) is to send them along with enough of their 'special' goodies to share around. Kids being what they are, their friends may well temporarily wish they were on the diet too, if only for the novelty of it.

ENTERTAINING AT HOME

One has to be just a little cautious about inviting even adult people for a meal. The snag lies in the fact that it will be extremely difficult for your guests to reciprocate by offering similar hospitality. Sometimes it is better merely to invite friends just for drinks or, if for an evening, then for 'coffee later on' asking them what time they can come after finishing their own evening meal. The only other alternative is to offer

INTRODUCTION 35

them dinner at a restaurant which you *know* can safely feed you. If they then wish to return that compliment, describe your problem to them and ask if they would mind booking at the same establishment, or some other which can cope in the same way.

If you have guests staying with you, or you particularly want to invite people to your own home for dinner, there is one important detail to consider. In our experience, while it is quite in order to provide one's guests with a few items of food which the arthritic person must not eat, one should be careful not to make the arthritic's diet look too different from that being offered to everyone else—or your visitors may somehow feel they are missing out on something special!

Again, let me stress the dangers to the arthritic of eating large quantites—and I say this with feeling, because it is when entertaining or in festive mood that I find myself most tempted to do so, or to bend the rules. Fatness is very bad for arthritis and, being human, ours is 'animal fat'—the very kind Dr Dong assures us we should not on any account take! If you think I'm being funny, just remember that having put on fat, you must again get rid of it for the sake of your joints, and the body does this by *absorbing* it. Painful joints and swelling may result, just as though you had eaten the fat, and will not ease out until your weight has stabilized once more. So do take care at all times.

TRAVELLING

Because we do a fair bit of getting about by road, and have found picnics in the driving seat less than ideal (sandwiches being fattening), it could get tricky if we failed to find a restaurant which was able to feed me. Since from time to time my job takes us all over Britain, in the end we sold our car

INTRODUCTION

and bought a modest motor-caravan, which solved all the problems. We can now cook and eat our own concoctions in peace and comfort, whenever and wherever we want. It may seem rather a drastic solution, but it does in fact suit our particular life-style very nicely—the only snag being the extra work for Judy!

When doing long journeys by rail or air, Judy usually makes me up an adequate supply of sandwiches. The average airline meal may just about produce a scrap of lettuce, and with luck a tiny roast potato or two which the gravy hasn't reached; but the chicken-breast is almost certain to have been treated with monosodium glutamate (to make it tastier, you know), and even that should therefore be avoided. So one sits munching sandwiches and getting the oddest looks. It can be most amusing, if you play it nonchalantly enough!

In foreign countries, enquire about the bread. Often it really will be made of only flour, water, yeast and salt—but do be perfectly certain it contains nothing else. The variety of available vegetables and fish is often far better than in Britain, and so long as the local wine has not been 'improved' by the addition of sulphur dioxide, and you stick preferably to a not too dry, white wine (the dry being more acid), you may find yourself feeding very well indeed.

So watch your weight. Which, before I hand over the book to Judy, brings me to some final words of advice:

TIPS ON 'CHEATING'

We all 'cheat' now and then when it comes to eating and perhaps drinking too, especially when the 'safe' varieties of goodies are limited, or there is simply nothing else available.

If you are really going to give Dr Dong's Diet a chance, however, it is essential *not to cheat at all* for at least the first fortnight, and preferably not even for the first month.

INTRODUCTION

One simply must give the thing time to set joints and muscles at ease first.

When you think you dare, a *small* diversion from the diet may be tried, but as the result is likely to make you sore . . . Well, put it this way; I always try to avoid eating anything doubtful unless I know for sure I have three clear days in which to be painful without it mattering too much. Why three days? For some reason, with me at least, it seems to take that amount of time, adhering strictly to the diet, to get right again after eating the wrong thing. And it can be *hell* for most of that time. So I would strongly advise that one should take extreme care not to experiment if you are about to travel, or have any important function or appointment lined up within the next few days.

After one has been on the diet for about a year, it is possible in some cases to get away with the occasional consumption of the 'wrong thing' without suffering excessively. In the early stages, however, my own bitter experience was that even the tiniest 'cheat', whether deliberate or accidental, was usually and *within the hour* more than quite enough to make me wish it hadn't happened. The pain of such reminders would invariably be with me for the best part of half a week. Even now, I consider it rarely worth even contemplating the risk. One develops very quickly a sort of conditioned mental reflex which (happily) makes doing without even the most particular of old favourites really no trouble at all.

Sometimes, of course, one has little alternative, as when given a meal by an acquaintance who doesn't understand (see p. 32). More often, however, it is a case of having tried something and found it did not in fact *seem* to cause you harm, because you may then be tempted to take more of whatever it was during the next few days as well—as when, for example, 'testing' a new brand of foreign margarine. With me, the trouble then creeps in gradually, so that only after some time am I aware that I am stiffening up, or moving more and more painfully. The toxic poisons have by that

INTRODUCTION

time built up to the danger level, albeit slowly, and it can then take every bit as long to rid one's system of them—once one has discovered and eliminated the cause.

Having explained in general terms how the diet works, and how I cope with it from day to day, I will let Judy give you more detailed advice and tell you of her excellent recipes in her own words.

May you now enjoy all the remarkable and wonderful relief which Dr Dong's Diet, and Judy's cooking, have given me; and in the prophetic words of my own doctor when I started on the diet: Good luck.

Putting the Diet into Practice

by Judy Andrews

I think the first thing I should say is that clearly it would be rather unfair to expect any non-arthritic members of the family to live entirely on this diet, just because one person in the household is doing so. There is no problem, however, because it is quite easy to cook a little meat for them at the same time as the dieter's food, and they can after all share the vegetables, even though these will have been produced without butter or pepper. My daughters are quite used to adding these things at table, as they know I will not have done so in the kitchen.

I do, all the same, have to be absolutely scrupulous about washing utensils with which foods unsuitable for Jim have been prepared. I also keep cooking oil used for frying things he must not have entirely separate from that which he and I use, as the merest trace of meat, tomatoes, etc., can cause him stiffness.

FINDING THE RIGHT FOOD

Finding food for people on Dr Dong's Diet does take a great deal of care. In Britain, however, we are fairly fortunate at present because there is, in any case, a general move towards natural, unadulterated food, usually termed 'Wholefood', and to organically grown vegetables.

I am often asked how I manage a busy life without all the usual 'convenience' foods. Of course I do use some of them, though only a few of the kind I normally bought before we

40 PUTTING THE DIET INTO PRACTICE

started on the diet. We have found a lot of interesting new ones (new to us, that is), and here a good health food store or counter can be of great assistance.

Although at first it might seem impossible to avoid monosodium glutamate and all those artificial colours, preservatives, flavourings and other chemical additives, one can nevertheless purchase quite a number of useful prepacked 'convenience' foods. You simply have to stop and read the label of every tin and packet and jar you pick up. And read it carefully! Often it is the last line or even the final word of the ingredients list which says 'flavouring', 'preservative' or 'colouring'. And one must be particularly cautious because as Jim has indicated on page 20, a manufacturer may change the ingredients in a product so that something once 'safe' may no longer be so.

This applies equally importantly to *any* food products you purchase. Take, for instance, soya sauce, peanut butter, salted nuts and potato crisps—to name but a few. Some brands are safely clear of, say, preservatives or other additives, while other makes *of the same thing* contain them for no very apparent reason, and are therefore unsuitable. Even though our recipes suggest soya sauce or whatever, it is of course up to the individual cook to check that the brand in use contains only permissible ingredients. What, then, does one do when one sees things like 'permitted colouring', or even unspecified 'vegetable colouring' (which might be fruit-based), on a label? We think it best to err on the safe side, and avoid taking unknown chances!

DO REMEMBER THAT EVEN THE TINIEST AMOUNT OF ANY OF THE ITEMS 'FORBIDDEN' IN DR DONG'S DIET MAY CAUSE YOU ACUTE DISCOMFORT, AND IT TAKES A LONG TIME FOR THE REACTION TO CLEAR AGAIN.

It is true that I spend more time cooking than I used to before we found Dr Dong's Diet, but many women I know who cook conventional things still spend far longer in their kitchens than I do even now. Some bake all the family's supplies of bread, cakes, pies and biscuits, as well as prepar-

PUTTING THE DIET INTO PRACTICE 41

ing three-course meals twice a day. So for many people, this diet may well mean less cooking, not more.

I realize that we are lucky that in our household the cook (me) is not the person with arthritic hands, and, to begin with, some people may find it physically impossible to manage some of the recipes I give. The point is that if you persevere with the diet, eating those dishes which are easier to prepare, the effects of it should enable you to do much more quite soon.

The following foods are those which we find particularly handy:

EGG-WHITE

A truly wonderful food, hygienically wrapped! Very quick to cook, versatile, rich in protein, and incredibly tasty. If you find it difficult to separate the white from the yolk, there are gadgets on the market which do this.

Throw away the yolk and shell. And if that sounds like sacrilege or wanton wastefulness, it isn't. If you accept this diet, the yolk must be considered as harmful—a poison, if you like —and discarded, just like the shell. However, if you can't bear to pour it down the drain, try digging it into a rose-bed if you have a garden. The roses won't waste it, believe me! I always imagined that most of an egg's flavour came from the yolk, but this really isn't so. A fried egg-white on toast makes an excellent breakfast dish, and Jim considers a poached egg-white better still. I do them for him in one of those cupped aluminium poaching dishes, greased with a smear of cooking oil. To do them in water in a saucepan requires the addition of vinegar, which 'isn't on', even in small quantities.

SWEETCORN

This useful product comes either tinned or frozen, on or off the cob. Whole cobs make a pleasant snack meal, or a grand 'starter' to a main course, the tinned ones being quicker to heat and often tastier, while 'cream style' corn can be used as a remarkably delightful sauce or pancake filling, and is

42 PUTTING THE DIET INTO PRACTICE

especially good in sandwiches. Sweetcorn soup (p. 76) is a firm favourite in our family.

TINNED FISH

Sardines or brisling make good luncheon dishes, either grilled on toast, or cold. The same applies to cod roe, pink or red salmon, tuna, mackerel, mussels, oysters, etc. These products can be particularly useful when one is travelling.

SALADS OF ALL KINDS

Well, what could be more convenient? Or better for you? Avoid tomatoes, though! Well-scrubbed tender young vegetables such as carrots make an excellent raw snack.

BREAKFAST CEREALS

As Jim mentioned earlier, the 'plain' ones like Rice Krispies Puffed Wheat, Cornflakes, Shreddies, Weetabix, and so on, may be found free of additives other than natural vitamins, and these, taken with plant 'milk' (see section on health food shopping below) can make a pleasant change now and then. Since these vegetable milks taste different from cows' milk, you may find a previously favourite breakfast cereal no longer goes well with what you now must take. We, for instance, find that Puffed Wheat, Shreddies and Weetabix go best with Plamil, but of course it's a matter for individual taste.

YEAST EXTRACT

There are several makes, of which Marmite is perhaps the best known, but do try a variety, as the flavours vary quite a lot. Yeast extract gives a superbly 'meaty' taste to a number of dishes, and stirred into very hot water makes a most acceptable 'instant consommé'. A large mugful is just the thing on a cold day.

Health Food Products

Health food shops have the advantage of being stocked with perfectly ordinary foods, some of which do not contain the usual additive 'cocktail' of ingredients. There is also quite a

PUTTING THE DIET INTO PRACTICE 43

surprising variety of different honeys to choose from, which, since jams, jellies and marmalades are 'out', is a boon.

The following items, which we have found particularly useful, can also be found in most health food establishments, as well as in an increasing number of ordinary grocery stores.

SOYA MILK
Such things as Plamil and Beanmilk (tinned, concentrated milk-like products made entirely from vegetable matter), are usually obtainable.

T.V.P.
Textured Vegetable Protein, mostly based on soya bean meal, and the various nut foods are a great attraction for the Dong Dieter. Both are meat-like in form, and so make a truly delicious change from seafood. But do look carefully at the packets, as some brands contain tomato or other unsuitable ingredients, like 'M.S.G.' (monosodium glutamate).

PROTOSE
A tinned savoury nutmeat, suitable for use in dishes which would otherwise be based on stewing beef.

PROTOVEG NATURAL FLAVOUR MINCED STYLE
This is textured soya protein in packets, and when reconstituted and flavoured with yeast extract, can be used as a substitute for minced beef as, for example, the basis of a succulent 'shepherd's pie'.

RISSOL-NUT SAVOURY NUT MIX
Also in packets, but contains only a little soya, its main ingredients being cashew nut and wheat. It makes extremely good sausages and rissoles.

PANTRY STOCK SAVOURY RISSOLE MIX
These convenient little packets make a good helping of very tasty rissoles for two people. It is very quick and easy to prepare, holds together well in the frying pan, and can be shaped into sausages if you prefer.

44 PUTTING THE DIET INTO PRACTICE

NUTTOLENE
A tinned 'luncheon meat', made from peanuts, cashew nuts and salt. Very good indeed with salads, or else sliced and grilled.

NUTTER
Yet another pure vegetable fat, to ring the changes.

PINTO BEANS
For those who had a passion for baked beans on toast, these taste surprisingly similar, even thought not in tomato sauce. Serve them the same way. Handy when you're in a hurry.

SWEETS
There are usually plenty of other goodies which can be enjoyed by people sticking to the diet. As a *very* occasional treat, one might try Granny Ann's Granymels, which are real, delicious caramels whose only bad effect seems to be the inevitable fattening one. (And don't be surprised if even a pound of extra weight starts hurting those arthritic joints.) Some arthritic people find they can eat carob, which tastes rather like chocolate; others experience subsequent pain.

BISCUITS
Allinson's makes a wide range of delicious sweet biscuits *some* of which are perfectly suitable for arthritics. We also use Barbara's 100% Whole Wheat Pretzels and Ideal Bran Thin Crispbread.

Fish

It's well worth seeking out a really good fish shop with plenty of variety on offer. Fishmongers in general are very helpful, and will usually say what is the best buy of the day. Be adventurous! You are going to be eating fish very frequently, so will appreciate the various flavours. Try anything the shop can provide; angler fish, sometimes

PUTTING THE DIET INTO PRACTICE   45

known as monkfish, is particularly delicious (so never mind what the beast looks like), and can be used to simulate several kinds of rather expensive shellfish, depending on how you treat it. I once made an extremely tasty meal from fresh saithe (called coalfish, or 'coalie' in some places), which the shop was selling fresh but very cheaply, expecting its customers to buy it for their cats!

Be very careful about smoked fish, which often contains colouring agents. An unusual orange tint will usually give the game away. The fishmonger may know of the 'safe' kinds, such as some Arbroath smokies, and Manx kippers. (The delectable Loch Fyne kippers are usually dyed, alas.)

When buying frozen fish, look carefully for an ingredients list on the package. So many makes contain monosodium glutamate, or other hazards. Most already breadcrumbed and 'battered' fish do. It is far safer to buy the plain things and bread or batter them at home. I find it most useful always to keep a bag of prawns in my freezer, as a tasty stand-by for the occasional unexpected guest.

The principal dangers when buying tinned fish are citric acid and tomato sauce, but tuna, salmon, cod roe, sardines and brisling are often free of these and other additives (olive oil is OK), as are certain brands of tinned shellfish, such as smoked mussels and smoked oysters, but *do read the list of ingredients*. Practically all the small jars of prawns, or potted goods, unfortunately, contain the very things one must avoid.

Don't assume that because one make of, say, tinned sardines is free from additives, all will be. They aren't, so beware!

Small tins of fish are especially useful when travelling, though those containing oil can present a disposal problem in trains and planes! If you have a car, I suggest you keep at least one tin of a fairly moist fish (pink salmon is ideal) and a packet of water biscuits or Ryvita in it for emergencies, together with a tin-opener and knife, of course.

Vegetables

Just as when buying fish, it is worth locating a really good supplier in order to get a wide range of varieties. As you will not require any fruit other than the occasional avocado 'pear', and in general because fish is cheaper than meat, you may well find you can easily afford to try some of the more unusual vegetables, such as Chinese cabbage and kohl rabi. Recently a far wider selection of imported produce has become available, from places all over the world, and one can have a lot of fun experimenting. And because with this diet we try to eat more than one kind of vegetable at a sitting, if one turns out less pleasant than expected, at least the entire balance of the meal is not spoilt.

Jim and I prefer not to eat potatoes every day, but rather regard them as just one of the many vegetables to choose from. In any event, it is important never to eat any green potato, as the green contains solanine, which is a poison. For this reason, all potato sprouts or shoots should be carefully cut away, along with any green parts, *before* cooking.

I consider rice to be less fattening than potatoes, and like to use brown rice, both for its better flavour and greater nutritional value. It is full of vitamin B, but it does take longer to cook, and is not so attractive on the plate.

Avocados are for us an occasional real luxury, though at certain times of the year they can be bought quite reasonably, especially when you consider that one feeds two people. They are normally served with a sauce containing acid, but are good on their own, simply cut in half and eaten with a teaspoon. (When guests are about, we fill the cavities with shrimps or prawns and top *their* helpings with mayonnaise.) Avocados are imported and mostly stored under light refrigeration, but will gradually ripen at room temperature. If very hard when you buy them, ripening may take several days. If held cupped in the hand and very gently squeezed, they will feel just soft when ripe, and by that stage some varieties have loosened the big stone inside, which can then be felt moving if you shake the fruit.

PUTTING THE DIET INTO PRACTICE   47

Nuts are a most useful source of protein and minerals. I often think vegetarians must find the many jokes about 'nut cutlets' rather puzzling. The Nut Roast on page 101–2 of our recipe section is especially delicious, either hot or cold. I usually serve it with poultry when we have guests, and invariably they take a second helping.

Margarine, Fats and Oils

Unlike British margarines which, apart from the Kosher Tomor, all seem to contain whey, some imported margarines, such as Vitaquell from West Germany, are milk-free. Certain additives are still likely to be present, however, so these goods should be tried with caution, and even if no pain is produced at once, used only occasionally.

Doctors tell us that 'saturated' fat is bad for our circulatory systems, and we should eat 'polyunsaturated' products whenever possible. Most animal fats, however, are saturated, as are some vegetable oils, such as coconut.

To make solid vegetable oils, manufacturers either choose a 'hard' or saturated oil, or else use a process called 'hydrogenization', which unfortunately reduces the polyunsaturates content.

The very best oils are 'cold pressed'. These are usually obtainable from health food shops, but tend to be expensive. Safflower oil is the richest of all in polyunsaturates, but it is somewhat difficult to find in Britain, and is rather costly.

Good, readily available oils for general use are corn oil, sunflower, soya bean, cottonseed and peanut. Sesame oil has a strong flavour which makes it less suitable for general use. Practically all vegetable oils can be considered 'safe' in Dr Dong's Diet, but some deteriorate when heated. Because corn oil does so to a lesser extent than others, I prefer it for most purposes, and usually buy it in five-litre cans from Boots.

Any oil which has been allowed to smoke should be discarded and not reused, since it has thus been made slightly poisonous.

48   PUTTING THE DIET INTO PRACTICE

For some purposes one does need a solid fat, and there are two main kinds available in Britain, which the Dong Dieter can use. These are pure solid vegetable oil (such as Pura), which is as hard as lard, and Trex, which has a creamy consistency. (I make up Jim's 'Vegerine' from one or other of the two—see p. 64.) There may well be other brands to look out for. The point is that in some cooking, a solid oil or fat produces a better final result than liquid oil, even if it has to be melted during the process. In others, a creamy substance such as Trex is best. In the recipes I have suggested in each case the product I have found most suitable.

Biscuits

Apart from the products available in health food shops (see p. 44) few biscuit manufacturers put a list of ingredients on their packets, and most of them mention 'shortening' without saying whether it is animal fat or vegetable oil. I never feel it is worth 'risking' these in Jim's case.

Most of the crispbreads (like Ryvita, for instance) are in fact 'safe', and we find that Carr's Table Water Biscuits are excellent and have no ill effects. Delice Pretzels (puff pastry decorative biscuits from West Germany) are also all right, and make a very pleasant change. Some health food stores stock a range of other perfectly 'safe' biscuits for this diet— but *do read the labels*.

PART TWO

RECIPE SECTION

Using the Recipes

ADAPTING ORDINARY RECIPES

While one can occasionally use T.V.P. in place of meat, most meat recipes cannot be altered sufficiently for the diet. A number of fish dishes, however, although unsuitable in the original state due to the suggested inclusion of lemon juice, tomato, or some kind of dairy product such as milk or butter, can be changed. If lemon juice or tomato forms an essential part of a recipe, there is little one can do, but where possible I simply omit them.

Egg-white is an even better medium for sticking bread-crumbs on to fish or other foods for frying purposes than a whole egg. For each egg in a recipe, I use either the white from one very large egg, or else the whites of two much smaller ones. In flavour or texture the lack of the yolk is rarely detectable, though where colour is concerned there is inevitably a slight difference.

Vegetable oil can be substituted for butter, margarine or lard in frying, sauces, etc., and water or vegetable stock can be used in place of liquid milk very successfully. Cheese must just be forgotten about, though those recipes which call for a sprinkling of cheese on top can often be done using a few breadcrumbs tossed in oil instead, and the dish browned under the grill. The result can be just as interesting.

In baking, the problem of replacement needs care. Sometimes hardened vegetable oils, such as Trex, can be used in place of butter, margarine or lard, but if you have to resort to liquid oil, remember that *only 3 fl oz (75 ml) of oil are required to*

USING THE RECIPES

replace every 4oz (100g) of solid fat. (2 tablespoons = 1fl oz or 25ml.) Replace half an ounce (12·5g) of flour in every 4oz (100g) with cornflour, and add an extra level teaspoonful of baking powder for every 4oz (100g), then sieve all the dry ingredients together and stir in the liquids, beating well.

Rum is a fair substitute for sherry in cooking. A little whisky or white wine can be used in dishes where other alcohol is called for.

GENERAL NOTES ON THE RECIPES

The recipes are to feed two people, as we find this handiest. It is not difficult to halve if you are on your own, or to put half away for tomorrow, and it is easy to increase quantities if need be.

Where I have said a 'teaspoon', this is always a *level* teaspoonful; if a heaped one is required, I have said so in the recipe. The same applies to 'tablespoon'.

To weigh syrup, I put the whole tin on to the scale, and remove the required amount. I call this 'weighing out'. It saves an awful mess, and is the only way I know to get an accurate amount of syrup.

'Flour' means *plain* flour. If self-raising is required, I have said so. I use wholemeal and 81% flours for most of my cooking, but this is a matter of taste. I also use brown sugars a good deal, as we prefer the flavour.

Except when quoting a friend's recipe, we have not used garlic as an ingredient because we personally do not like it. However, it is excellent nutritionally, so there is nothing wrong with adding it, or any other herb, wherever you fancy a more piquant flavour.

Caution! As both of us have already stressed, putting on weight is disastrous for arthritic people, so do eat sparingly and infrequently of the more fattening things such as pasta, fries, puddings, cakes, and so on. The only reason we have included any such recipes, is that we think everyone is entitled, just once in a while, to have a go at something different as a special treat.

Bon appétit!

Drinks, Hot and Cold

When taking tea without milk, you may find you prefer a weaker brew. We like China tea, and vary our choice between Lapsang Souchong (which has a slightly smoky flavour), Keemun, and Jasmine tea, in which the dried jasmine flowers give a delicately fragrant aroma and smoothness. We are also fond of the Ceylon (Sri Lanka) brand, Poonakandy. These and many other teas can be purchased in teabag form, or loose, but it is still necessary to *read the ingredients list*, as some teas do contain 'flavouring' unspecified.

Coffee, both ground and instant, can be taken 'black'. Jim and I drink decaffeinated instant coffee with our breakfasts and at mid-morning, but sometimes percolate ground coffee as a luxury in the evening.

As already mentioned, a teaspoonful of yeast extract stirred into a mug of very hot water makes an extremely pleasant drink for a really cold day.

Most health food shops supply a choice of other hot drinks, usually made from a variety of grains and herbs. We like Postum very much, as it has some of the 'body' of a milky drink.

Bottled soft drinks and squashes all contain fruit and/or additives, so soda water seems to be the only harmless soft commercial drink you can buy, though gentle experimentation with natural 'spa' waters may provide further alternatives.

Commercial vegetable juices usually contain tomato, or chemical additives, and if you have a 'juicer' you can make your own. We discovered a real liking for carrot juice, which

DRINKS, HOT AND COLD

is rich and sweet, but must be freshly made. We have had some success with combinations such as carrot and parsnip but, in general, juicing can work out very expensive, simply because it takes a large quantity of the vegetable in question to produce a small amount of juice. For us it is a 'once in a while' drink, and makes a special treat.

Jim has found that he can get away with taking just the odd glass of white wine (but *not* red) with a meal without ill effect, though if he does so on several successive days, he does get a bit achy. Not everyone on the diet can take it though, so if you like wine, we would suggest waiting until you have completed at least a month following the diet to the letter, without wine, before trying a very small glassful.

An occasional and very small Scotch whisky, rum, or even vodka, will probably cause little harm *if well diluted*. The last two can both be made more interesting by the addition of a leaf or two of mint or balm, or a slice of cucumber, and some ice. Jim has found it best to avoid altogether any drink (other than additive-free white wine) which is based on grapes or any other kind of fruit.

Commercial beer, to Jim's sadness, is mostly right out of the question, because of additives in almost all tinned, bottled, keg, and even 'Home-Brew' kinds. Being so fattening, it is best avoided anyway. Commercial ginger-beer is usually laced with chemicals, but fortunately a most acceptable and easily made home-brewed ginger-beer is possible, and becomes very 'smooth' indeed when made to the following recipe and allowed to mature for a few months. It is excellent added to rum or vodka.

A Ginger-Beer 'Plant'

Powdered yeast
Water
Sugar
Ground ginger

DRINKS, HOT AND COLD

Dissolve 2oz (50g) yeast in ½pt (250ml) water in a largish container. Add 2 teaspoons of sugar, and 2 teaspoons of ground ginger. Feed this 'plant' with 1 teaspoon of ginger and 1 teaspoon of sugar each day, for 7 days.

On the 8th day, gently pour or siphon just the 'clear' liquid off the top of the sediment into a large bowl or a bucket. It is important to avoid including any of the yeasty sediment, as if even a tiny amount gets into the bottles, the latter may eventually explode inconveniently.

Add 4 pints (2.3 litres) of cold water.

Warm a further 2 pints (1 litre) of water in a pan, and in this dissolve 1¾lb (800g) of sugar. Add this syrup to the mixture in the bowl (bucket) and stir. In all, this now amounts to about 7 pints (4 litres).

Decant into *strong* screw-cap bottles, leaving a good air-space in each. Close tightly, and store in a cool place for at least 2 weeks before drinking (longer is better). Chill bottle before opening, to avoid over-effervescence.

If you wish to continue production, add 1 pint (0·5 litre) of cold water to the original sediment, and mix thoroughly. While it is still cloudy, divide it into 2 separate containers, and feed both of these new 'plants' at once—or throw or give one away. Repeat process above.

Mint Julep

> 1 teaspoon sugar
> ½ wineglassful water or soda water
> 3–4 sprigs of fresh mint
> 2 *small* glasses whisky

Put sugar, water or soda water, and mint, into a large bowl and stir well, until the flavour of the mint is extracted.

Add the whisky.

Fill tumblers with crushed ice and pour the julep over, decorating with sprigs of mint.

Breakfast Dishes

Some commerical breakfast cereals have additives in them other than the usual vitamins, and must therefore be avoided by Dong Dieters, but some are perfectly good. Read the ingredients lists carefully.

In place of milk, you can use soya 'milk' such as Plamil or Beanmilk, or even carrot juice.

For porridge, and other tasty hot breakfast dishes, see below.

Toast or bread can be given a thin smear of 'Vegerine' (p. 64), and a little honey, ginger-spread, or our Marrow and Ginger Preserve (p. 64–5).

Porridge

> 1 part rolled oats
> 3 parts water
> Pinch of cooking salt

Put oats and water in a pan and bring slowly to the boil, stirring a good deal. When boiling, add salt to taste.

Turn down the heat, and simmer for at least 5 minutes. If the porridge then looks too thick, add a little water and bring back to the boil, stirring well. (Taken without milk, porridge needs to be more 'liquid' than the normal consistency.)

Oaty Nosh

> 1 part oil
> 4 parts rolled oats
> 1 part soft brown sugar

58   **BREAKFAST DISHES**

Warm oil in frying pan. Sprinkle in the oats, and turn continually with a fish-slice, until they begin to brown.

Sprinkle with sugar. Turn for another minute, then serve in a cereal bowl and eat while still warm.

Egg-White Omelet

> *For each person:*
> 1 tablespoon sweetcorn kernels (or chopped mushrooms etc.)
> 2 teaspoons vegetable oil
> 2 egg-whites
> Pinch of cooking salt

Prepare the vegetables, and sauté lightly in the oil, in an omelet pan. (A non-stick frying pan will do, though the real thing is better. I recently bought a grand little Teflon-coated omelet pan from Woolworth's—one doesn't have to 'go expensive'!)

Meanwhile place the egg-whites in a roomy bowl with the salt. Remove the vegetables from the pan, using for preference a perforated spoon, and add them to the egg-whites. Stir this mixture gently—*do not beat.*

Pour the mixture back into the pan, which should not have been removed from the heat, and sauté until lightly browned underneath. Turn and cook the other side, then serve at once. (It is best to cook each individual helping separately, as omelets rarely benefit from being kept warm.)

Poached Egg-White

We suggest using a proper 'egg poacher'. Place a little water in the lower part, and bring to the boil. Lightly smear the cup of the upper part with cooking oil.

Separate the egg, and put the white into the upper part, with a pinch of salt added if desired. Poach for a few minutes until the white has gone opaque, but only just 'set'.

Serve on toast smeared with a little 'Vegerine' (p. 64).

BREAKFAST DISHES

Scrambled Egg-White

For this you will want at least 2 egg-whites per person. Put a knob of Trex or similar vegetable fat into a small pan, and melt it on a low heat. Meanwhile separate the eggs, and stir the whites together in the pan until they have turned solid white.

Serve on hot 'Vegerined' (see p. 64) toast.

Fried Egg-White

Fry the white in Trex or vegetable oil exactly as if it was a whole egg. You may find you prefer it slightly crisper round the edges than before.

Baking Breads and Scones

Yeast Bread

$\frac{3}{4}$ pint (375 ml) water
3 teaspoons dried yeast, or 1 oz (25 g) fresh yeast
1 x 25 mg vitamin C tablet
2 teaspoons sugar (white or soft brown)
2 teaspoons cooking salt
1 oz (25 g) Trex (vegetable fat)
1½ lb (700 g) flour (white, brown, granary, or wholemeal)

Bring water temperature to 110°F (43°C). If you have no cooking thermometer, do this by adding ¼ pint (125 ml) boiling water to ½ pint (250 ml) of cold. Into this hand-hot water stir the yeast, the crumbled vitamin C tablet, and 1 teaspoon of the sugar. (If using dried yeast, set this mixture aside to become frothy, for about 10 minutes, before proceeding.) Meanwhile dissolve the salt and the remaining sugar in the rest of the water.

Rub the Trex into the flour in a large bowl.

When the yeast mixture is ready, add both liquids to the flour in the bowl, and mix to form a firm dough, then turn it out on to a floured surface and knead it vigorously for 10 minutes. If you are unable to manage this, an electric mixer fitted with a dough-hook works almost as well if left mixing for at least 8 minutes. If you can do it by hand, though, really bash the dough—it's a grand way of letting off steam! (The exercise will help strengthen arms and wrists.) If dough has been insufficiently kneaded, the resulting bread will have

BAKING BREADS AND SCONES 61

huge holes in it, and be crumbly. One can hardly knead for too long.

Either shape the lump of dough and place it in a 2 lb (1 kg) loaf tin, or divide it into two and place in two 1 lb (500 g) tins. Alternatively shape it into 2 'cobs' on a baking sheet (or 1 cob and 6–8 small rolls). Cover with a clean teatowel, and set in a warm place to rise.

If you have no suitable 'warm place' (such as beside a solid-fuel fire or wood-burning stove), dough will in fact rise at room temperature, or even in a domestic refrigerator if you wish to retard it for some reason. It will take about an hour in a warm place, or 2–3 hours at room temperature, or up to 24 hours in a fridge.

A handy 'warm place' can be simply made by laying an insulated food-box on its side, and placing the loaf tins inside it together with a few jars of hot water. The average insulated food-box holds a 2-lb loaf tin and 4 coffee jars of hot water.

While the dough is rising, pre-heat the oven to a very high temperature, 500°F (240°C) Gas Mark 9. When the dough has *doubled its size,* turn the oven down to 450°F (230°C) Gas Mark 8, and put the bread in the centre of it. Bake for 45–50 minutes for a 2 lb loaf, or 30–40 minutes for 1 lb loaves or 'cobs', and 15–20 minutes for rolls.

To find out if the bread is ready, free it from the tin using an oven cloth, turn it over, and tap the base. If it sounds 'hollow', it's OK.

Leave it to cool on a wire rack.

Note: Bread freezes very well. When it has cooled, the loaf can be put into a polythene bag, and the air sucked out of the bag with a drinking straw before it is sealed. Frozen bread will keep for up to a year in a four-star freezer. Then, when it is required, allow it to thaw at room temperature, or else pre-heat the oven to 320°F (170°C) Gas Mark 3, wrap the bread in foil and cook for 10 minutes.

BAKING BREADS AND SCONES

Soda Bread

This kind of bread is extremely popular in Ireland, where it is often cooked in flat farls on a griddle. (The word 'farl' comes from Ancient Norse—a relic of Viking invasion—meaning a quarter; hence our old 'farthing', a quarter of a penny.)

Any plain flour is suitable for this recipe, though wholemeal does not rise as much as white flour, so a mixture of half wholemeal and half white makes a really lovely, tasty loaf. Ordinary self-raising flour is not good, being made from too 'soft' a wheat for bread. In some places however one can buy special 'soda bread self-raising flour' which is of course ideal.

To make a plain-flour soda bread loaf, you need:

> $1\frac{1}{2}$ lb (700 g) flour
> $1\frac{1}{2}$ teaspoons cooking salt
> $\frac{3}{4}$ teaspoon bicarbonate of soda
> $1\frac{1}{2}$ teaspoons cream of tartar
> About $\frac{3}{4}$ pint (375 ml) cold water

Sift together the flour, salt, bicarbonate of soda and cream of tartar. Then use a metal spoon to mix in the water quickly and lightly, adding just sufficient to give a soft, but not sticky, dough.

Turn the dough out on to a floured surface and shape it into a long cake. This can be baked in a 2 lb (1 kg) loaf tin, or on a baking sheet, in a hot oven, 450°F (230°C) Gas Mark 8, for 50 minutes.

SODA FARLS

Use half the above quantities, and shape the resulting dough into a disc about $\frac{1}{2}$ in (1 cm) thick, and cut this into quarters. Bake the quarters on a hot, lightly greased griddle (or thick-based frying pan) until the first side is nicely browned (in about 5–7 minutes), then turn them over and complete the cooking.

BAKING BREADS AND SCONES 63

Scones

 8oz (225g) self-raising flour (or 8oz plain and 3 teaspoons baking powder)
 ½ teaspoon cooking salt
 4 tablespoons vegetable oil
 5–6 tablespoons water

Mix all the dry ingredients together, and stir in the oil and water. Mix thoroughly to form a soft dough.

Knead the dough lightly, then roll to ½in (1·5cm) thick. Cut into rounds, placing these on a greased baking tray. Bake in a hot oven, 450°F (230°C) Gas Mark 8, for 10–12 minutes.

These can be eaten with 'Vegerine' (p. 64) and honey, or a ginger-spread. If sweeter scones are preferred—and they're pretty fattening anyway, so beware!—add 1 heaped teaspoon of castor sugar or soft brown sugar and, if you like, 1–2oz (25–50g) of finely chopped preserved ginger.

Spreads

'Vegerine'

In place of butter or margarine on bread, we use two kinds of spread, and refer to either under the heading of 'Vegerine'.

The easier one to make is that using Trex (pure vegetable fat), beating it until it is smooth and creamy, and then adding in a little salt, and beating it again. About ½ teaspoon of salt, to a 250 g (8·82 oz) packet of Trex seems about right.

If Trex is not obtainable, I buy solid vegetable oil, which in Britain comes in 500 g (1·1 lb) packs. Melt this down on a gentle heat, then stir in 2–3 tablespoons of liquid vegetable oil, such as corn oil, and put it aside to set again. If you can catch it while it is half set, you can beat in a little salt, which improves it.

Neither kind of 'Vegerine', as made above, has much of a flavour to it, but it does, as it were, 'lubricate' bread or toast, in much the same manner as margarine or butter.

Marrow and Ginger Preserve

To each 1¼ lb (600 g) prepared vegetable marrow, add:
1 lb (500 g) sugar
1 teaspoon ground ginger
1 small piece of stem ginger, bruised

Prepare the marrow by cutting it into thin slices, peeling them, and removing the seeds and pith, then chopping into small dice. Place these in a large pan with some of the sugar sprinkled over them, and leave for at least 1 hour.

By the end of this time, a quantity of clear juice will have

SPREADS 65

run from the marrow. Add the remaining sugar and both kinds of ginger to the pan, and bring it slowly to the boil, stirring. Continue to boil until all the marrow has become translucent, stirring it very frequently.

Meanwhile set the jars to warm. You will need about 1–2 jars per lb (500 g) of sugar.

Remove the stem ginger, and either liquidize or pass the marrow through a pureé-maker or a sieve. Return it to the pan, and bring back to the boil. Then pot it quickly, and seal.

If using transparent jam-pot covers, I like to soak these in cold water, shake off surplus drops before placing them over the jar, and then put on the elastic band while the 'jam' is still very hot, pulling the top smooth. When the 'jam' cools, a partial vacuum is formed inside the top, ensuring a good seal.

Note: This spread is not a true jam, as it contains no fruit pectin or gelatine, and thus does not set like a jam.

First Course Dishes

Mixed Hors-d'Oeuvres

This makes an excellent starter if you are entertaining, as you can include for your guests things which the arthritic person does not eat. It can be prepared well in advance, and arranged attractively on individual plates, or in an hors-d'oeuvres dish. The secret of a really good mixed hors-d'oeuvres is contrast—in shapes, colours and flavours. We suggest a selection from the following:

> Tinned sardines, brisling, or anchovies
> Lettuce, bean-sprouts, spring onions
> Parsley (dense heads on short stalks)
> Celery (cut in short lengths)
> Radishes, grated raw carrot, Chinese cabbage
> Cucumber (diced or thinly sliced)
> Beetroot (either grated raw, or cooked and sliced or diced)
> Shrimps or prawns (cooked and peeled)
> Sliced hard-boiled eggs (these can be included so long as the arthritic person knows only to eat those bits without the yolk)

For those who are not arthritic, one can serve real mayonnaise, and fruit- or mango-chutney, in separate bowls. The arthritic person can have a small separate helping of the Special Salad Cream (p. 158).

See also Samphire, on page 146.

If you have a copy of *New Hope for the Arthritic* by Dr Dong and June Banks, do try their Gado Gado on page 207 of that

FIRST COURSE DISHES

book. It is a delicious Indonesian dish, akin in a way to a mixed hors-d'oeuvres.

Avocado with Prawns

    1 ripe avocado pear
    Prawns or shrimps
    Parsley to garnish

Halve a really ripe avocado, and remove the stone. Fill the cavity in each separate half with prawns or shrimps, and serve on a lettuce leaf.

An alternative filling could be tinned tuna, or salmon, and a little parsley goes well as a garnish.

Avocado Supreme

    1 avocado pear
    1 tablespoon of soya sauce
    1 small carrot

Halve the avocado lengthwise, and remove the stone. Scoop out the flesh into a small bowl, add the soya sauce, and mash together using a fork.

Replace the mixture in the 'shells' of the avocado skin, and place under a hot grill for 5 minutes. Garnish quickly with a sprinkling of finely grated raw carrot, and serve at once.

Tastes absolutely fantastic!

PÂTÉS

I feel that pâté always looks best when served on individually prepared plates, which is anyway most convenient when entertaining. This can be done in advance, and decoratively set out before people come in for the meal. Plates can be made pretty by putting some lettuce leaves on each one, with a knob of pâté in the centre, and a small salad

FIRST COURSE DISHES

of cucumber slices, grated beetroot or carrot, mustard, cress, or parsley, and any other available salads, arranged around it. Fingers of thinly cut brown bread or toast are the traditional accompaniment.

Tuna Pâté

>   3½ oz (99 g) tin of tuna fish
>   Trex (vegetable fat)
>   Soya sauce

Open the tin and pour the oil off the tuna fish. Empty the flesh into a bowl and mash it vigorously with a fork. Add a small knob of Trex, and a dash of soya sauce, and beat well. Taste the mixture, adding more Trex or sauce if required.

The pâté can be served on small biscuits or squares of toast to make canapés or a savoury, or used as an excellent sandwich filling.

Granose 'Sandwich Spread'

This wonderfully tasty commercial product is a truly excellent vegetable pâté in its own right. We suggest serving it like any traditional pâté. Your guests are sure to be most impressed.

Aubergine Pâté

>   1 aubergine
>   Salt
>   Olive oil
>   Ground nutmeg

Halve the aubergine, sprinkle with salt, and cook it in the oven until the skin is black. Scoop out the flesh and mash it very thoroughly with some oil and a little salt and nutmeg. Taste, and adjust the seasoning. Serve in the traditional manner.

FIRST COURSE DISHES

69

Smoked Fish

Many kinds of fish can be smoked and served as a starter. Salmon, eel, trout, mackerel, mussels, all smoke well. Arrange them attractively on lettuce on individual plates, served with fingers of brown bread. (We include an interesting Chinese recipe for home-smoking on pp. 85–6).

Smoked mussels can be bought in tins containing nothing harmful to the arthritic, and are very good—for instance with lunch on small family celebrations.

Egg 'Mayonnaise'

If you have visitors, you can serve them the normal egg mayonnaise of hard-boiled eggs, halved, and placed sliced-side down on lettuce, then coated with ordinary mayonnaise.

The arthritic person can enjoy an almost identical dish simply by first removing the yolk from the halves of hard-boiled egg, omitting the mayonnaise, and coating the eggs instead with some of our Special Salad Cream (p. 158).

Stuffed Vine Leaves

> 1 small onion
> 1 tablespoon vegetable oil
> 2 tablespoons long-grain white rice
> 1–2 tablespoons flaked almonds
> 7 oz (198 g) tin of tuna fish
> Pinch of chopped mint (fresh or dried)
> Pinch of cooking salt
> Pinch of cinnamon
> 10 young vine leaves
> A little white wine, if liked

Chop the onion finely, and then fry gently in the oil for a few minutes. Add the rice, and continue to cook very gently until it is a pale golden colour. Add the flaked almonds, and reheat for just one minute, before removing the pan from the

FIRST COURSE DISHES

heat to add the tuna, mint, salt, and cinnamon. Stir well.

Bring a large pan of water almost to boiling, and dip the vine leaves in it for a minute, just to make them flexible. Remove them with a perforated spoon, and drain them well. Spread them out flat, and place a tablespoonful of the tuna mix on to each one, then fold them up carefully to make neat little envelope-style parcels.

Arrange the parcels gently in the bottom of a saucepan, and cover them with water, or a mixture of white wine and water. Bring slowly to the boil, cover the pan, and simmer for about 25 minutes, then remove the lid and continue cooking until almost all the liquid has gone.

Serve either hot or cold.

Note: If vine leaves are unobtainable, small cabbage leaves make a most acceptable substitute!

Soups

Vegetable stock, the water in which any vegetable has been boiled, contains many useful vitamins and minerals, and therefore should not be discarded without good reason. It can be used for making soups and sauces, and even for boiling the next vegetable. Some stock, such as onion, adds a marvellous flavour to sauces.

I do not keep the stock from cauliflower, or from Jerusalem artichokes, as I find these tend to induce uncomfortable flatulence. This also applies to the water used to soak or cook dried beans.

Instant Consommé

> Vegetable stock or water
> Yeast extract

This is most useful, as it can be made quickly. Heat stock or water until just slightly hotter than you like your soup to be. Put a teaspoonful of yeast extract into a mug or soup bowl. Pour on the water, and stir until the yeast extract is fully dissolved.

Yeast extracts vary in flavour. By experimenting with brands, you are sure to find a favourite taste—and the best amount to use each time.

Quick Fish Soup

This is a Chinese-style soup, which takes about 15 minutes to prepare.

72 SOUPS

$\frac{3}{4}$ pint (375 ml) fish or vegetable stock, or water
1 very small onion, or $\frac{1}{4}$ medium onion
$\frac{1}{4}$ lb (100 g) filleted white fish
2 teaspoons cornflour
1 teaspoon rum
2 teaspoons soya sauce
1 teaspoon yeast extract
$\frac{1}{4}$ teaspoon cooking salt

Put the stock or water on to boil, and cut the onion into small pieces. Add these to the boiling water and simmer for 10 minutes.

Meanwhile, cut the fish into bite-sized chunks. Mix 1 teaspoon cornflour with the rum and 1 teaspoon soya sauce in a small bowl, and stir in the fish until it is well coated. Set aside.

After the 10 minutes of simmering, add the yeast extract and salt to the pan. Dissolve the remaining cornflour in the rest of the soya sauce, and add this to the pan as well. Return the contents to the boil, stirring, and add the pieces of fish. Cook for only 2 minutes, and serve at once.

Watercress and Fish Soup

This Chinese-style soup tastes strangely like artichoke.

2 oz (50 g) white fish
1 teaspoon rum
1 teaspoon cornflour
Pinch of cooking salt
2 oz (50 g) watercress
1 pint (500 ml) fish or vegetable stock, or water.

Remove any skin or bones from the fish and chop the flesh into tiny pieces.

Mix together the rum, cornflour and salt. Add the chopped fish, stir well, and leave to marinate for at least 20 minutes.

SOUPS

Wash the watercress and chop it coarsely. Pieces should not exceed ½ in (1 cm).

Just before the soup is needed, boil the stock or water and add the fish and watercress. Return to the boil and simmer for 2 minutes. Serve at once.

Thick Fish Soup

½ pint (250 ml) fish or vegetable stock, or water
¼ pint (125 ml) soya milk
2 oz (50 g) mushrooms—stems will do for this
2 oz (50 g) white fish
2 teaspoons cornflour
Pinch of cooking salt
2 oz (50 g) frozen peas

Reserve 1 tablespoon of stock or water, putting the rest into a pan with the 'milk'. Bring to the boil. Chop the mushrooms finely and add these to the pan. Simmer for 15 minutes.

Meanwhile, remove any skin and bones from the fish and chop the flesh into very small pieces. Mix the cornflour to a smooth cream with the stock you reserved, and add a pinch of salt to the mixture.

After the 15 minutes of simmering, add the cornflour, fish, and peas to the pan, and return to the boil, stirring all the time, and cook for 3 minutes. Taste, adjust the seasoning and serve at once.

Doris's Fish Soup

This very delicious recipe was given to me by a Maltese friend. Any fish can be used, but the oilier types, such as herring, mackerel, and salmon, are not as suitable as other kinds.

½ lb (200 g) fish
1¼ pints (625 ml) water
1 large carrot
1 clove of garlic or a good pinch of garlic granules

74 SOUPS

    1 tablespoon vegetable oil
    1 small onion
    6 mint leaves, finely chopped
    2 big sprigs of parsley, finely chopped
    ¼ teaspoon cooking salt

If using whole fish, discard the guttings. Cut into 3 or 4
pieces. Put the flesh, skin and bones into a pan with 1 pint
(500 ml) water and boil for about 20 minutes. Sieve it, retain
the stock, and discard the fish.

Meanwhile peel and slice the carrot and put into ¼ pint
(125 ml) water and boil until soft. Make them into a purée,
using either a liquidizer, or a purée-maker, or by mashing
them as best you can with a fork.

Slice and fry the garlic in the oil until it is soft; add the
onion, finely chopped, and when it begins to soften, add the
chopped herbs. (If using garlic granules, add them to the
onion with the mint and parsley.)

Finally, mix together the fish stock, the carrot purée and
the garlic, onion, salt and herbs.

Reheat, and serve.

Mushroom Soup with Egg-Whites

    ¼ lb (100 g) mushrooms
    Handful of watercress, parsley or spring onions
    1 pint (500 ml) vegetable stock or water
    2 teaspoons soya sauce
    2 egg-whites

Chop the mushrooms and greens roughly. Add them to the
stock or water, and simmer until they are tender.

Add the soya sauce, and then very carefully slide in the
egg-whites. Poach gently, until the whites are ready. Serve.

SOUPS

French Onion Soup

> 3 medium onions
> 2 tablespoons vegetable oil
> 1 pint (500 ml) vegetable stock or water
> ½ teaspoon yeast extract
> 1 bayleaf
> Cooking salt
> 1 teaspoon cornflour

Peel and finely chop the onions. Fry very gently in the oil until they become golden and soft. Add the stock or water, and the yeast extract and bayleaf, and simmer for 15 minutes.

Remove the bayleaf and taste the soup, salting it as required. Thicken it with the cornflour dissolved in a little cold water. Bring back to the boil stirring, and serve very hot.

Vegetable Broth

This is a handy soup, as it can be made with any vegetables that are available. Small quantities of different things make it especially interesting. All vegetables should be cut, diced, grated, etc., so that there are no large pieces.

> 2 pints (1·1 litre) vegetable stock or water
> ½ pint (300 ml) mixed vegetables
> 1 oz (25 g) barley
> ½ teaspoon yeast extract
> Cooking salt

Put the stock or water on a high heat. When it is boiling, sprinkle in the barley and vegetables. Stir in the yeast extract, and bring back to the boil. Reduce the heat and simmer gently, with a lid on the pan, for at least 2 hours.

Taste, salt as necessary, and serve.

Cream of Beetroot Soup

1 small onion
2 tablespoons vegetable oil
¾ pint (375 ml) vegetable stock or water
½ lb (200 g) sliced cooked beetroot
Cooking salt
Ground nutmeg

Peel and slice the onion, and fry it gently in the oil until it is thoroughly soft, then pour off as much of the oil as possible.

Add the vegetable stock or water, and the beetroot. Bring to the boil, then simmer for 30 minutes.

Liquidize thoroughly, then reheat, taste and season with salt and ground nutmeg. Serve at once.

Note: This soup is a very striking colour. If you swirl a little undiluted soya milk into each bowl just before serving, it becomes positively spectacular!

Cream of Sweetcorn Soup

1 onion
2 tablespoons vegetable oil
12 oz (340 g) tin of sweetcorn kernels
1½ pints (850 ml) vegetable stock or water
Cooking salt

Peel and finely chop the onion, and sauté it gently in the oil for about 5 minutes, without letting it brown. Add the sweetcorn and the stock or water, then bring to the boil and simmer for 30 minutes.

Remove a good ladleful of this, and set it aside. Liquidize the rest thoroughly. Return to the pan, and add in the ladleful, thus giving some texture to the soup. Add salt to taste, reheat and serve.

SOUPS 77

Cream of Mushroom Soup

$\frac{1}{4}$lb (100 g) mushrooms
$\frac{3}{4}$ pint (375 ml) vegetable stock or water
1 tablespoon vegetable oil
1 tablespoon flour
2 parsley stalks
Cooking salt

Wash and slice the mushrooms, and if large, cut the slices in half. Put into a pan with the stock or water; bring to the boil, and simmer for 10 minutes.

Using a sieve, drain the mushrooms, reserving both mushrooms and stock.

Warm the oil in a large saucepan, stir in the flour, and cook gently until this 'roux' bubbles, then beat in the mushroom liquid. Add the parsley stalks, and simmer for about 10 minutes.

Remove the parsley stalks, add salt to taste, and return the mushrooms. Cook for about 3 minutes, to heat thoroughly.

This soup looks most attractive served with croutons, or a swirl of undiluted soya milk.

CROUTONS
Cut a slice of bread into small dice, about $\frac{3}{4}$in (1·5 cm) square, and fry to a golden brown in a little vegetable oil.

Cream of Parsnip Soup

$\frac{3}{4}$lb (350 g) parsnips
1 carrot
1 onion
1 bayleaf
2 tablespoons vegetable oil
$1\frac{1}{2}$ pints (850 ml) vegetable stock or water
Ground mace or nutmeg
Cooking salt
Chopped parsley or spring onion to garnish

Peel and chop the parsnips, carrot and onion. Sauté them with the bayleaf in the oil for 10 minutes, without browning. Add the stock or water, and cook for 45 minutes.

Remove the bayleaf, and liquidize the soup thoroughly. If it is for immediate use, season with mace or nutmeg and salt, then reheat and serve. If not, set it aside, or freeze it, and when it is required, reheat it, season, and serve. Garnish with chopped parsley or spring onion.

Note: This soup freezes particularly well.

Spinach Soup

> 1 onion
> 1 tablespoon vegetable oil
> ½lb (200g) fresh spinach or a small packet of frozen
> ¾ pint (375ml) vegetable stock or water
> Cooking salt
> Ground nutmeg

Peel and chop the onion, and fry gently in the oil for 5 minutes. Pour off as much oil as possible. If using fresh spinach, wash it well and chop roughly, then add the stock or water, and the spinach, to the onion in the pan. Frozen spinach may be either thawed in advance, or added direct to the pan. Bring to the boil, and simmer for 15 minutes.

Liquidize this well, then add salt and ground nutmeg to taste. Reheat and serve. A little undiluted soya milk may be swirled into each bowl for pretty effect.

Main Course Fish Dishes

Poached Fish

Poaching is a grand way of cooking all fillets of white fish, such as cod, haddock, whiting, plaice or sole.

In a suitable ovenproof dish, arrange a bed of vegetables like onions or mushrooms, or merely grease the dish. Lay the fillets on top, either flat or rolled up, and pour over them vegetable stock or water. Bake in a moderate oven, 350°F (180°C) Gas Mark 4, for about 20 minutes.

If you have used a bed of vegetables, this should be carefully drained, and served along with the fish. The stock can be used to make a tasty white sauce.

Foil-Baked Fish

This method is suitable for any fish, whole, filleted or in steaks. Cut a generous piece of foil for each separate piece, and wipe it with a little vegetable oil. Lay the fish on the foil, and if you like spread on it a suitable vegetable mixture, such as fried onions and peas, or sweetcorn kernels, or stuff whole fish with a vegetable, breadcrumb and herb mixture moistened with an egg-white. Make the foil into a loose parcel, and place the parcel(s) on a baking sheet.

Bake in a moderately hot oven, 375°F (190°C) Gas Mark 5. Fillets will only require about 25 minutes, but a big whole fish such as a salmon or a sea-trout (salmon-trout) may take an hour or more. Test by opening the top of the parcel and prodding the fish with a skewer to see if it is tender.

Grilled Fish

Most fish are suitable for grilling, either whole, filleted, or cut into steaks.

Line the grill pan with foil, wipe the foil with vegetable oil, and lay the fish carefully on to it. Wipe the top surface of the fish with oil. Using a medium-hot setting, with the fish not too near the heat, grill until the flesh of the fish no longer has a raw transparent look.

Thin fillets will not need turning. For thick fillets, steaks, or whole fish, turn once. Cook the less attractive side first, so that you do not have to turn a second time when dishing up. Lift the fish very carefully on a fish-slice.

It cooks very quickly, so all vegetables should be almost ready before you start grilling the fish itself. If it has time to get over-cooked, it will be chewy, and the flavour will be spoilt.

Fried Fish

Frying is suitable for all filleted fish. It can be fried without any coating, but this tends to make a rather oily dish, which is unnecessarily fattening. If you do not want to coat the fish, it will probably be better to grill it.

There are two methods which I find satisfactory: shallow frying, coated with egg and crumbs, or deep frying in batter.

SHALLOW FRYING

Prepare the fish carefully, removing any bones, cutting off any raggy bits, and drying the fish well on absorbent paper. Dip into salted flour, then into lightly beaten egg-white, then into a plate of crumbs.

Suitable crumbs can be made by putting Weetabix into a liquidizer, and running it at slow speed. Several other 'harmless' breakfast cereals, such as cornflakes, can be used in the same way.

Egg-white on its own actually sticks crumbs on to fish better than whole egg does.

MAIN COURSE FISH DISHES 81

Fry the crumbed fillets in about ½ in (1 cm) of vegetable oil, for a few minutes. (About 5–6 minutes is right for most fillets.) Then turn, and cook on the other side. Fillets should be put into the oil skin-side up first, so that when turned they are the right way up for serving. Dish them up straight away, when ready.

Again, all vegetables should be almost cooked before you fry the fish.

DEEP FRYING

Prepare the fish as for shallow frying, but instead of dipping them into flour, dip into batter (see below), and at once slip them into deep fat, which should be good and hot, at 375°F (190°C) if you have a thermostat or thermometer for your deep-fat pan. Cook until the batter is a rich golden colour.

BATTER

> 3 tablespoons flour
> ½ teaspoon baking powder
> ¼ teaspoon cooking salt
> Cold water

Sift the dry ingredients together into a basin, and mix to a coating consistency with cold water—when the consistency is right it will coat the back of the spoon you mix it with.

Fish Pasties

This is an 'idea', rather than a recipe; any fish can be used, cut into small pieces, and any vegetable also cut into small dice. Large pasties can be served as a main course; small ones as a starter or snack, and tiny ones as canapés with drinks. Pasties also make an ideal cold picnic lunch, or can be kept hot in a wide-necked vacuum flask.

Make some pastry (shortcrust or flaky, see p. 166–7). Gather together other suitable ingredients, such as diced fish, or shellfish, diced root vegetables, chopped 'greens',

82 MAIN COURSE FISH DISHES

sprigs of cauliflower, peas, sweetcorn, chopped hard-boiled egg-white, or whatever you fancy.

Make a white sauce, using vegetable oil, flour and any well-flavoured stock or water. Stir in the fish, vegetables and egg-whites.

Roll out the pastry, and cut it into rounds. Put a suitable quantity of the fish mixture on to each round, fold over and seal.

Cook on an oiled baking sheet in a hot oven 425°F (220°C) Gas Mark 7, for about an hour.

Serve hot or cold. For a picnic we wrap the pasties in foil, then in a clean cloth (teatowel), to retain the heat as long as possible.

Fish Casserole

This is suitable for any white fish like cod, haddock, plaice, sole, whiting, etc.

    Potatoes
    1 small onion
    7 oz (175 g) white fish
    ½ pint (250 ml) water
    1 tablespoon vegetable oil
    2 tablespoons flour
    Cooking salt

Peel potatoes until you have about ½ lb (250 g) prepared. Boil them, and slice thinly.

Chop the onion, and poach it and the fish in the water for 10 minutes. Drain, retaining the water. Flake the fish, and carefully remove any bones and skin. Arrange the flaked fish and onion in an ovenproof dish.

Heat the oil in a small pan; stir in the flour with a wooden spoon and cook until it is frothy. Stir in the fish stock, and cook until it is a smooth, thick sauce. Taste, season and pour the sauce over the fish.

Cover the top of the casserole with sliced potatoes, and

MAIN COURSE FISH DISHES

brush with a little vegetable oil. Grill for 3–5 minutes, and serve very hot.

Fish Crumble

This is suitable for any white fish: cod, haddock, plaice, sole, whiting, etc.

> 6oz (150g) white fish
> ¼ pint (125ml) vegetable stock or water
> 3 tablespoons oil
> 2 tablespoons flour
> ½ level teaspoon yeast extract
> Cooking salt

Poach the fish in the vegetable stock or water for 10 minutes, then flake it, removing any skin or bones. Retain the stock.

Warm 1 tablespoon of oil in a small saucepan, stir in 2 tablespoons flour with a wooden spoon, and cook until it froths without allowing it to brown.

Gradually blend in the stock, and when it is hot, stir in the yeast extract and cook the mixture, stirring continuously until it boils and thickens. Simmer for 2 minutes, stirring to give the sauce a good 'polish', then stir in the fish. Add salt to taste. Pour this into an oiled, 1 pint (500ml) ovenproof dish.

To make the crumble, mix the remaining flour with the remaining 2 tablespoons of oil, and sprinkle this thickly over the fish mixture. Bake in the centre of a moderately hot oven, 375°F (190°C) Gas Mark 5, for 25–30 minutes, or until the crumble is golden.

A most popular dish.

Stuffed Cabbage Leaves

Cod or haddock are the best for this dish, but any other white fish will do.

> 1 small onion
> 1 tablespoon vegetable oil

MAIN COURSE FISH DISHES

6 large cabbage leaves
2 tablespoons flour
$\frac{1}{2}$ pint (250 ml) vegetable stock or water
$\frac{1}{2}$ lb (200 g) fish

Put a large pan of water on to boil. Meanwhile, chop the onion and fry it very gently in the oil.

Plunge the cabbage leaves into the boiling water for 1 minute. Remove them with a perforated spoon, drain, and set aside.

Sprinkle the flour into the oil and onion, and stir it with a wooden spoon until it froths, then add the vegetable stock or water and bring to the boil, stirring all the time. Reduce the heat, and continue cooking gently.

Cut the fish into bite-sized pieces, and stir into the sauce. Cook for 3 minutes, then put a sixth of the mixture into the centre of each cabbage leaf. Fold into tidy parcels, and place these in a suitable ovenproof dish, which should be oiled. Add a little water, cover the dish with a lid or some foil, and bake in a fairly hot oven, 400°F (200°C) Gas Mark 6, for 15 minutes. Lift the parcels on to a clean dish, and serve hot.

Chinese-Style Fish

1 tablespoon cornflour
1 tablespoon soya sauce
1 tablespoon rum
2 tablespoons fish or vegetable stock, or water
1 tablespoon molasses
$\frac{3}{4}$ lb (350 g) white fish
1 small onion
Vegetable oil
Additional vegetable stock or water as required

Mix the cornflour, soya sauce, rum, 2 tablespoons stock or water, and molasses, in a generous-sized bowl. Cut the fish into bite-sized pieces, and stir them in. Leave to marinate for $\frac{1}{2}$–3 hours, stirring occasionally.

MAIN COURSE FISH DISHES 85

Slice the onion, and fry it gently in a little vegetable oil until soft. Meanwhile put the fish into a sieve over a bowl, to drain.

Add the fish to the onion, and continue to fry gently for about 5 minutes, turning frequently.

Add more water or stock to the cornflour/soya sauce mix, and stir well. Add this to the pan, and continue to stir until it has thickened. If it seems too thick, add some more liquid.

Cook for a few minutes more, then serve very hot, with boiled rice.

Smoking Fish the Chinese Way

Any fish may be smoked, having first been prepared and then marinated overnight. Smoke it in the oven—in a well-ventilated kitchen!

Marinade for 2 good-sized fish fillets
3 tablespoons soya sauce
1 tablespoon rum
2 teaspoons finely chopped onion
2 teaspoons ground ginger

Smoking Mix
2 oz (50 g) sugar
2 oz (50 g) Indian tea leaves

Note: For a pair of small whole mackerel or trout, double the marinade ingredients.

Make the marinade by mixing together the soya sauce, rum, onion and ginger. Fillets need no preparation, but whole fish should be scored on both sides. Place in the marinade overnight, or for a minimum of 12 hours.

Line a baking tin with foil, and sprinkle in the sugar and tea. Put this into a hot oven, 425°F (220°C) Gas Mark 7.

Arrange the marinated fish on an oiled wire rack. As soon as the sugar and tea mixture is smoking vigorously, put the

MAIN COURSE FISH DISHES

rack of fish over it, and reduce the oven temperature to moderately hot, 375°F (190°C) Gas Mark 5. Smoke for about 20 minutes for a whole trout, or 15 minutes for haddock fillets.

Serve either hot, or else cold with salad.

Hairy Tatties

This is a traditional Scottish dish, made from dry-salted cod.

$\frac{1}{2}$lb (200g) salt-cod
3 medium potatoes
1 tablespoon olive oil

Soak the fish in cold water for 24 hours, changing the water twice during that time.

Next, place the fish in fresh cold water, in a saucepan, and bring to the boil, boiling for 30 minutes. Pour off this water, and leave the fish to cool.

Peel the potatoes, cut into small pieces, and boil in unsalted water until soft. Mash.

Remove the skin and bones from the fish, and break the flesh into small flakes. Take a fork or a wire beater, and beat the flakes into the potato, then add the oil, and beat very well again, until the fish is broken up into fine 'hairs' (hence the name).

The dish is now ready, but for extra effect, it can be put into an oiled pie-dish and baked in a moderate oven, 350°F (180°C) Gas Mark 4, until the top is golden.

Serve hot, with green vegetable.

Haddock Bake

This is an excellent dish for using up stale bread. (Brown bread makes the tastiest topping for it.)

8oz (200g) haddock
Fish or vegetable stock, or water
1 tablespoon vegetable oil

MAIN COURSE FISH DISHES 87

2 tablespoons flour
Cooking salt
Breadcrumbs

Put the haddock into a pan, covering it with stock or water. Bring to the boil, then remove from the heat. Allow to stand for 10 minutes before carefully draining the stock from the fish, retaining both. Flake the fish, removing skin and bones.

Heat the oil in a small pan, stir in the flour, and cook until it froths, then add some of the stock and cook until it thickens. If necessary, add more stock, or some water, to make a thick sauce. Taste, and salt it if you think it's needed.

Gently stir the haddock into the sauce, and put the mixture into an oiled ovenproof dish.

Mix together some breadcrumbs and enough oil just to moisten them all. Put a layer of this mixture over the top of the dish, and place the whole thing under a hot grill, until the top is crisp and golden.

Serve hot.

Kedgeree

4 tablespoons long-grain rice (brown or white)
Cooking salt
8 oz (200 g) Finnan haddock (or other undyed smoked haddock)
2 eggs
4 oz (100 g) peas
Vegetable oil

Cook the rice in plenty of boiling water with some salt. White rice will take only 15 minutes to soften; brown is very variable, but takes a good deal longer.

Place the fish in a pan, and cover with cold water. Bring it slowly to the boil, then remove from the heat, put a lid on the pan, and leave for 10 minutes to cook the fish. Drain the fish and flake it up, discarding skin and all bones.

Put the eggs into cold water, bring to the boil and boil for

MAIN COURSE FISH DISHES

10 minutes. Pour off the water, crack the eggshells, and cover with plenty of cold water. When cool enough to handle comfortably, shell the eggs, cut in half, remove and discard the yolks, and cut the whites into small pieces.

If using fresh peas, cook them in boiling water until tender. If using frozen peas, drop them into boiling water and turn the heat off. Stand for 3 minutes, then drain the peas.

Warm some oil in a saucepan, and put in the rice, fish, peas and egg-whites. Stir all together, taste, and add extra salt if needed. Continue to turn the kedgeree over a medium heat for about 5 minutes, but add extra oil if it sticks. Ensure it is warmed right through, and serve very hot.

Note: Other vegetables can be used instead of, or as well as peas.

Fried Herring

> 2 small herring
> Cooking salt
> Oatmeal
> Vegetable oil

Prepare the herrings by cutting away heads, tails and fins. Clean and wash the fish, and open them out to remove the backbones. Sprinkle with salt. Put them together, skin outwards, and dip in oatmeal. Fry in a little oil for 7 minutes, then drain and serve.

Stuffed Herring or Mackerel

> 2 fish
> 2 oz (50 g) fine oatmeal
> Pinch of cooking salt
> Chopped celery leaves, parsley and chives
> 1 tablespoon vegetable oil

MAIN COURSE FISH DISHES 89

Clean the fish. Mix the remaining ingredients together well, and stuff the fish sparsely with the mixture. (The oatmeal will swell during cooking.) Bake in an oiled baking tin in a moderate oven 350°F (180°C) Gas Mark 4, for 40 minutes, basting occasionally.

Baked Mackerel

Prepare the fish, which must be very fresh, by removing the head, tail and fins. Line a baking tin with foil smeared with a little oil, and lay the fish inside. Sprinkle with salt, and bake in a hot oven, 425°F (220°C) Gas Mark 7, for about 25 minutes.

Baked Stuffed Mackerel

> 2 mackerel
> Brown breadcrumbs
> Chopped celery leaves
> Chopped parsley
> Vegetable oil

Remove head, fins and tail from the mackerel, then open them and remove the backbone.

Make the stuffing by mixing breadcrumbs with a little chopped celery and parsley.

Place each fish on a generous-sized piece of foil, which should be lightly oiled. Fill with the stuffing, and close them up. Make loose parcels with the foil and place these on a baking sheet in a fairly hot oven, 375°F (190°C) Gas Mark 5, for about 25 minutes, until the fish are tender.

Poached Stuffed Mackerel

> 2 mackerel
> 4 tablespoons fresh brown breadcrumbs
> 2 teaspoons fresh, or 1 teaspoon dried, chopped tarragon

MAIN COURSE FISH DISHES

1 tablespoon runny honey
Chopped parsley to garnish

Prepare the mackerel as for baking. To make the stuffing, mix together the breadcrumbs, tarragon and honey. Fill the fish with the stuffing, and fold them up. Place in a suitable ovenproof dish, and add a little water. Poach in a fairly hot oven, 375°F (190°C) Gas Mark 5, for 35 minutes.

Serve sprinkled with chopped parsley.

Salmon Cakes

$7\frac{1}{2}$oz (213g) tin of salmon
3 egg-whites
3 tablespoons finely chopped onion, or 2 tablespoon dried onion
$\frac{1}{2}$ teaspoon cooking salt
Breadcrumbs
Vegetable oil

Drain the tinned salmon, remove dark skin and bones, and mash the flesh with a fork. Add the egg-whites, onion and salt. Beat well, then allow the mixture to stand for at least 5 minutes.

Add breadcrumbs gradually until the mixture is thick enough to form into flat cakes. Fry these in the oil until they are nicely browned on both sides. Serve at once—they are superb!

Trout with Almonds

An impressively tasty dish, grand for entertaining.

Court Bouillon
1 pint (500ml) water
1 onion
1 carrot

MAIN COURSE FISH DISHES

1 stick of celery
Bouquet garni
$\frac{1}{4}$ pint (125 ml) white wine, if desired

A trout for each person

For every 2 trout:
1 tablespoon olive oil
1 oz (25 g) flaked almonds
$\frac{1}{4}$ teaspoon cooking salt
Watercress or parsley to garnish

First make the bouillon, placing all the ingredients except the wine in a pan and simmering for 30 minutes. Strain, and allow to cool, then add the wine if it is being used.

Wash, dry, and trim the trout, leaving their heads on. Arrange them in an ovenproof dish, cover with the bouillon, and poach in a very cool oven, 225°F (110°C) Gas Mark $\frac{1}{4}$, for 15–20 minutes. When the fish are cooked, their eyes will have whitened.

Once the fish is almost ready, heat the olive oil in a small pan; add the almonds and cook slowly until toasted to a pale golden brown. When the trout is done, remove it from the oven, drain (retaining the stock to make a sauce tomorrow), and carefully remove the skins and heads. Arrange the fish nicely on a serving dish, and keep warm.

Sprinkle the salt on to the almonds, and pour them and their oil over the fish. Serve at once, garnished with watercress or parsley, or surrounded by green peas.

Tuna Hot-Pot

This makes an excellent dish if you have to be out for a few hours before a meal. It is forgiving. It tastes much more like a meat dish than a fish one, and the flavour is surprisingly reminiscent of Lancashire Hot-Pot!

1 onion
1–2 carrots

3–4 potatoes
7oz (198g) tin of tuna
Cooking salt
Water

Peel and slice the onion, and spread the slices in the bottom of a casserole. Peel and slice the carrots and potatoes (enough for 2 helpings). Arrange half the potatoes over the onions, and place the carrot slices over the potatoes.

Open the tin of tuna, and pour off the oil into a small bowl. Break up the fish and spread it in a layer over the carrots. Sprinkle with salt to taste.

Arrange the remaining potato slices in a very tidy layer over the fish, and thinly pour the tuna oil carefully over all of them. Add water to about half-way up the food.

Bake in a moderately hot oven, 325°F (170°C) Gas Mark 3, for about 2 hours. This can then be served as it is, or first browned under the grill.

Angler Fish 'Scampi'

$\frac{1}{2}$–$\frac{3}{4}$lb (200–350g) angler fish (monkfish)
1 or 2 eggs
1 or 2 weetabix 'biscuits'
Vegetable oil

Cut the fish into pieces the size and shape of large prawns. Separate the eggs (1 large or 2 small eggs should give you sufficient white) and beat the whites lightly.

Crush the Weetabix into fine crumbs, or liquidize it to that effect.

Dry the fish, dip it into the egg-white, then into the crumbs, and fry it quickly in hot, deep oil.

Serve as for scampi—the texture and taste are so similar to the real thing, you'll hardly know the difference!

Main Course Shellfish Dishes

Prawns and Vegetables, Chinese-Style

> 1 small onion
> 2 Brussels sprouts
> 1 small carrot
> 1 small parsnip
> 1 stick of celery
> 4 tablespoons long-grain rice (brown or white)
> 2 teaspoons cornflour
> 2 teaspoons runny honey
> 1 tablespoon soya sauce
> About $\frac{1}{4}$ pt (125 ml) vegetable stock or water
> 1 tablespoon flaked almonds
> Vegetable oil
> 1 tablespoon frozen peas
> 1 tablespoon frozen sweetcorn kernels
> 2 oz (50 g) prawns (fresh or frozen)

Prepare all the vegetables. Peel the onion and cut it into quarters; peel the sprouts and cut into quarters; peel the carrot and slice diagonally; peel and dice the parsnip; remove any 'strings' from the celery stick, and slice it across thinly.

Cook the rice in plenty of boiling water. If using white rice, it will require about 15 minutes. Brown rice takes a good deal longer, some types needing almost 45 minutes, but it is better, tastier, and more nutritious than white.

Put the cornflour, honey and soya sauce into a cup. Add 2 tablespoons of the stock or water, and stir all together well. Stand this aside.

Just 15 minutes before the mealtime, you can start to cook. First fry the onion and almonds in some vegetable oil for 5

94   **MAIN COURSE SHELLFISH DISHES**

minutes, then add all the remaining vegetables, and stir-fry for a few minutes. Add the prawns, and continue stirring. Now pour in the rest of the stock or water, and bring it to the boil. Stir the cornflour mix, and add it to the pan, and continue cooking, still stirring, until the whole thing is hot, and the sauce has thickened.

Serve hot, with rice.

Note: Vegetables may be varied, as available, but try for a wide selection of colours, shapes, and flavours.

Prawns in Dragon Sauce

This dish is specially designed for prawns which have roe clustered on them, and is most attractive and tasty.

>About 12 fresh prawns with roe
>Chopped tarragon (fresh or dried)
>¼ pint (125 ml) fish or vegetable stock, or water
>1 tablespoon oil
>2 tablespoons flour

Scrape the roe carefully off the prawns into a small bowl, shell the prawns, and put them in a separate container. Put some tarragon in a third bowl, and pour the hot stock or water over it. Leave it to infuse and cool.

Cook the prawns for 3–4 minutes in a little boiling water.

Make a thick sauce by warming the oil, adding the flour and cooking until it froths, then adding the tarragon stock, and stirring vigorously, until it has thickened. If it is too thick, add a little of the water in which the prawns were cooked. Stir the prawn roe into the sauce. When the eggs touch the hot sauce, they will become bright red. Stir in the prawns, and serve hot.

Shrimp or Prawn Flan

>*For the pastry*:
>8 oz (200 g) plain flour

MAIN COURSE SHELLFISH DISHES 95

½ level teaspoon cooking salt
4 oz (100 g) Trex
Cold water

For the filling:
Shelled shrimps or prawns
Sweetcorn kernels
Peas
3 egg-whites
4 fl oz (100 ml) fish or vegetable stock, or water

First make the pastry by sieving the flour and salt into a bowl, and rubbing in the Trex. When all the Trex is completely rubbed in, stir in a little water, using a metal knife. Add just enough water to form a very stiff dough. Roll this out on a floured board, and line a flan dish or ring.

Fill the flan with prawns or shrimps, and vegetables. Make a 'custard' by beating together the egg-whites and the stock or water, and pour this carefully over the fish and vegetables.

Bake in a moderately hot oven, 375°F (190°C) Gas Mark 5, for an hour.

Serve warm or cold. This makes a really delicious picnic dish.

Shrimp or Prawn Soufflé

¼ lb (50 g) shelled shrimps or prawns (fresh or frozen)
3 tablespoons vegetable oil
2 tablespoons flour
½ pint (250 ml) fish or vegetable stock, or water
Cooking salt
4 egg-whites

If using frozen prawns or shrimps allow them to thaw completely before starting to make this dish. In an emergency this can be done in moments by tossing them into a little boiling water, and using this water as part of the stock.

96 MAIN COURSE SHELLFISH DISHES

Warm the oil in a roomy saucepan, stir in the flour and cook until it froths. Stir in the stock or water and cook, stirring, until the sauce thickens. Stir in the shellfish, taste, and add salt as required. Allow this sauce to cool a little.

Whisk the egg-whites very stiffly, then fold them into the prawn (shrimp) sauce. Pour the mixture into a greased 2-pint (1-litre) soufflé dish or ovenproof dish, and bake in a moderately hot oven, 400°F (200°C) Gas Mark 6, for 45 minutes. Serve quickly before it sinks!

Pink Pasta

3–4 oz (100 g) spaghetti or macaroni
1 tablespoon diced raw beetroot
¼ pint (125 ml) mixed vegetables (peas, sweetcorn, broad and runner beans, diced carrot, diced parsnip, etc.)
1 medium onion
1 tablespoon vegetable oil
2 tablespoons flour
½ pint (250 ml) vegetable stock or water
A good handful of shelled prawns or shrimps (fresh or frozen)
Soya sauce
Cooking salt

Boil the pasta, beetroot and the mixed vegetables, in a large pan of water until the pasta is cooked, and all the vegetables are tender. (Pasta is ready if when broken or cut it has no white core.)

Meanwhile, chop the onion, and fry it in the vegetable oil until it is soft. Stir in the flour and cook until it froths. Add the stock or water, and continue to stir until the sauce thickens. Add in the shellfish and a dash of soya sauce. Taste, and add more soya sauce or some salt as necessary.

Drain the pasta, and serve, with the sauce mixture poured over it.

Unusual, and rather pretty.

MAIN COURSE SHELLFISH DISHES 97

Mussels in Vegetable Sauce

Mussels can be purchased either fresh or frozen. Fresh ones must be alive, with their shells tightly closed; frozen ones are sold without their shells.

To prepare fresh mussels, scrub them very well, and rinse them in at least three changes of water to remove any grit or mud. Then scrape the shells with a knife to remove the filament, and lift the shells out of the water leaving the filament behind.

> 16–25 mussels, according to size
> $\frac{3}{4}$ pint (375 ml) vegetable stock or water
> $\frac{1}{4}$ pint (125 ml) chopped vegetables (onion, celery, carrot, etc.)
> Bouquet garni
> Cooking salt
> 2 tablespoons vegetable oil
> 2 tablespoons flour
> Parsley to garnish

If using fresh mussels, put them into a pan with the stock or water, the vegetables, the bouquet garni and a little salt. Bring to the boil, and continue to cook. As the shells open, lift out the mussels on a perforated spoon, leaving the stock simmering, and remove the mussels from their shells.

If using frozen mussels, bring the stock, or water, vegetables and bouquet garni to the boil, then dip the mussels in the boiling stock for just 1–2 minutes, remove and set aside.

Keep the mussels in a covered dish while preparing the sauce, to prevent them from drying up.

When the vegetables are tender, remove the bouquet garni from the pan, strain the stock and add the vegetables to the mussels.

Make a sauce by warming the oil, stirring in the flour, and cooking until it foams. Then add in $\frac{1}{2}$ pint (300 ml) of the stock, and bring this to the boil, continuing to stir. Go on cooking it until it is properly thickened and well polished.

98 MAIN COURSE SHELLFISH DISHES

Finally, stir the mussels and vegetables into the sauce, cook for a few minutes longer, and serve very hot, garnished with parsley.

Casserole of Scallop

Fresh or frozen scallops can be used for this dish. Fresh ones are in season during the late winter and spring. Wash them well, and use the white and bright orange portions. Frozen scallops can be used without thawing.

> 4 large or 8 small scallops
> Fish or vegetable stock, or water
> Pinch of cooking salt
> 2 tablespoons vegetable oil
> 2 tablespoons flour
> $\frac{1}{4}$ level teaspoon dry mustard
> 1 level teaspoon yeast extract
> 2 tablespoons fresh breadcrumbs

Put the scallops into a pan, cover with stock or water, and add a pinch of salt if the stock is not already salted. Bring slowly to the boil; cover the pan, and lower the heat to poach for 7 minutes.

Lift the scallops out with a perforated spoon, and drain them on kitchen paper. Cut them into 1-in (2.5cm) pieces, and arrange in an oiled, shallow, heatproof dish.

Measure $\frac{1}{4}$pt (125ml) of the poaching water, and if there isn't enough of it, add more stock or water to make up this amount.

Warm 1 tablespoon of the oil in a small saucepan, stir in the flour and mustard, and cook for 2 minutes, stirring. Do not allow it to brown. Blend in the poaching water, and cook, still stirring, until the mixture comes to the boil and thickens. Simmer for 3 minutes.

Remove from the heat, and stir in the yeast extract until it is fully dissolved. Taste the sauce, and add salt if required. Pour the sauce over the scallops.

MAIN COURSE SHELLFISH DISHES 99

Mix together the breadcrumbs and the remaining tablespoon of oil, and sprinkle over the scallops and sauce.

Cook for 10–15 minutes towards the top of a hot oven, 425°F (220°C) Gas Mark 7. Serve hot.

Main Courses Without Fish

POULTRY

Jim found that when he was first on the diet even a little of the white meat of turkey or chicken caused him some discomfort, but after six months he tried again, and discovered that it was now just about all right—so long as he really took very little.

If the arthritic person in your household is to be able to try a little roast turkey or chicken, and also its stuffing, these must *not* be cooked together; the juices for the wrong parts of the bird will invade the stuffing during cooking.

Instead of a stuffing I make a Nut Roast (pp. 101–2) and cook it in the oven at the same time as the bird. Jim then serves spoonfuls of this along with the meat, and guests invariably talk of the 'lovely stuffing', and come back for second helpings. Frankly, I find a turkey dinner an excellent way of feeding a large party—at *any* time of the year—and Jim's fondness of the accompanying nut roast, in this case made with chestnuts, prevents him from being tempted into eating too much of the meat!

Note: If the bird has been frozen, it is *most important* to be absolutely sure it is thoroughly thawed before attempting to cook it. Medium-sized chickens may take up to 12 hours, while turkeys may need up to 48 hours, at room temperature. To make certain all is well, push your hand into the body of the bird; if it feels any colder than the room outside it, then it is not completely thawed. If you cook it too soon, you run the risk of getting salmonella—a particularly dangerous form of food poisoning.

MAIN COURSES WITHOUT FISH 101

Roast Turkey

Heat the oven to 425°F (220°) Gas Mark 7. Prepare the bird by plucking any feathers which have been left on, and then rubbing some vegetable oil into the skin of its breast and legs.

Peel 1–2 potatoes, and put them into the body of the bird, where they will steam during cooking, so keeping the flesh nice and moist. Place the turkey in a roasting tin, breast uppermost. Do not cover the tin.

Cook in the centre of the oven, basting frequently during cooking. After $1\frac{1}{2}$ hours, test to see if it is cooked by pricking the flesh with a skewer—if the juices run clear, the bird is ready. A small turkey takes about $1\frac{1}{2}$ hours; a bird over 14 lbs (6·5 kg) will need up to 2 hours. This may seem an unusually short cooking time, but using such a high oven temperature for a brief period like this, does produce delicious results.

Roast Chicken

Try to obtain a chicken which has not been caponized or injected with something to 'improve' its meat.

The most satisfactory method of roasting chicken I know is to use a roasting bag, following the instructions on the packet (these vary a bit with the different brands, but the results seem much the same with any I have tried).

I normally massage some vegetable oil into the skin of the bird before sliding it into the bag, to make it go crisp and brown in the cooking. I happen to like it that way, though Jim avoids eating the skin for arthritic reasons.

Nut Roast

This delicious dish is an excellent main course, hot or cold, and can be made with any kind of nuts, or a mixture of several sorts. The character of the finished flavour depends on the variety one has used. A chestnut roast, for instance,

MAIN COURSES WITHOUT FISH

has a marvellously 'Christmassy' flavour, and is a perfect accompaniment to roast turkey. Note that peeling and chopping chestnuts can take a *very* long time!

½lb (200g) chopped nuts
1oz (25g) fresh brown breadcrumbs
1 small onion
1 tablespoon cooking oil
2 tablespoons wholemeal flour
½ pint (250ml) water
Pinch of cooking salt
½ teaspoon yeast extract
1 egg-white

Mix the nuts and breadcrumbs together in a large bowl.

Peel and chop the onion and fry in the oil until soft, then stir in the flour and cook until it froths. Add the water and salt, stirring until it is warm, then add the yeast extract and continue stirring until this is fully dissolved, and the sauce has thickened.

Mix the sauce into the nut mixture, add the lightly beaten egg-white, and beat all together well.

Pour the mixture into an oiled loaf tin, and bake in a moderately hot oven, 375°F (190°C) Gas Mark 5, for 30–40 minutes.

'Protoveg' Hot-Pot

This is, in fact, extremely like an Irish Stew.

1 medium onion
2–3 potatoes
5oz (142g) sachet of Protoveg 'Chunky Style, Natural Flavour'
Vegetable oil
1 teaspoon yeast extract

MAIN COURSES WITHOUT FISH 103

Vegetable stock or water
Cooking salt

Peel and chop the onion. Peel the potatoes and slice fairly thickly. Put the onion into the bottom of a deep, ovenproof dish, and cover it with a sparse layer of potato slices. Sprinkle on half or all of the Protoveg—the diameter of your dish will decide if you should make one or two layers; if making a second layer, it should be divided from the first by another sparse layer of potato slices. Top with a good layer of potato, carefully arranged, and brush this layer with vegetable oil.

Dissolve the yeast extract in a little of the liquid. Add this to the casserole, and top up with stock or water to just below the top layer of potato, adding salt to taste.

Cook in a warm oven, 325°F (170°C) Gas Mark 3, for 2 hours. If you like the top browned nicely, you can raise the temperature to hot, 425°F (220°C) Gas Mark 7, for the last half-hour, or put the dish under a hot grill for a few minutes just before serving.

When dishing out, make sure you dig right down to the bottom of the dish for each helping, so that everyone gets some of the onions.

Shepherd's Pie

2–3 medium potatoes
Cooking salt
1 teacup Protoveg 'Natural Flavour, Minced Style'
1½ teacups vegetable stock or water
2 teaspoons yeast extract
1 tablespoon vegetable oil
A little soya milk

Peel the potatoes, cut them into small pieces and boil in salted water until soft.

Meanwhile, hydrate the Protoveg by putting it into a small saucepan with the stock or water, the yeast extract and the

MAIN COURSES WITHOUT FISH

oil. Bring this to the boil, and simmer for 3 minutes. Put it into an oiled ovenproof dish.

When the potatoes are ready, drain them and mash with enough soya milk to make a creamy mashed potato. Spread this over the Protoveg; roughen the surface with a fork, and cook in a moderately hot oven, 375°F (190°C) Gas Mark 5, for half an hour.

Quick 'Protose' Nosh

2 large onions
Vegetable oil
½ parsnip
1 carrot
1 tablespoon yeast extract
¼ pint (125 ml) water
1 tin Protose
1 tablespoon frozen peas
1 tablespoon frozen sweetcorn

Peel and slice the onions, and fry them gently in some vegetable oil in a roomy frying pan. Grate the parsnip into the frying pan, and continue to fry, turning occasionally, while you peel the carrot and slice it thinly (if the slices are large, they should be cut into quarters). These can then be added to the contents of the pan.

In a small saucepan, dissolve the yeast extract in the water, and bring to the boil. Add this to the frying pan, bringing back to the boil, and simmer gently, stirring now and then.

Open the tin of Protose and cut the contents into rough dice. Add these to the vegetables, and continue stirring occasionally until the Protose becomes warm and soft, then add the peas and sweetcorn and simmer for 3 minutes before serving.

MAIN COURSES WITHOUT FISH 105

'Nuttolene' Fritters

6 slices of Nuttolene about $\frac{1}{2}$in (1 cm) thick
2 rounded tablespoons flour
1 teaspoon baking powder
Pinch of cooking salt
Cold water
Vegetable oil

Cut the Nuttolene into slices.

Make a batter by sifting the flour, baking powder and salt into a bowl, and beating in the water gradually, until it is smooth and will coat the back of a wooden spoon.

Dip the Nuttolene slices into the batter, and fry in deep oil until a rich golden brown.

Serve at once.

Savoury Fritters

1 tablespoon flour
Pinch of cooking salt
2 egg-whites
A filling, such as sweetcorn, peas, shrimps, etc.
Vegetable oil

Sift the flour and salt into a bowl. Add the egg-whites, and beat until a smooth batter is formed. No further liquid is required. Stir in a suitable filling, such as the contents of a 7 oz (198 g) tin of sweetcorn, or a large handful of frozen peas or shrimps.

Heat a frying pan with a little oil in it, and put tablespoonfuls of the batter into it, well spaced out. Fry until brown, turning once. Serve hot. If you are using sweetcorn as a filling, an accompanying green vegetable looks nice.

Pancakes

These are what my mother calls a 'pan-to-plate' meal. Get

MAIN COURSES WITHOUT FISH

everyone sitting at the table before you start to cook, and serve each one as it comes off the pan. This way you get the best of the flavour.

4 oz (100 g) plain flour
½ teaspoon cooking salt
2 egg-whites
½ pint (250 ml) vegetable stock or water
Vegetable oil

Sift the flour and salt into a bowl, make a 'well' in the centre of it, and add the egg-whites and the stock of water. Beat all very well together, until there are no lumps, using a whisk or wooden spoon. Allow this to stand for at least half an hour before starting to cook it.

Prepare the filling, and keep it warm before making the pancakes.

Use a small frying pan or omelet pan. Heat the pan with only a little oil, pour in a thin layer of batter, and fry this until the underside is lightly browned and there is no liquid batter left. Then, either turn the pancake, cook its second side, and fill and eat it at once, or, if you wish to keep the pancakes for a while, do not cook the second side, but instead make a pile of them as they are, on a plate. When cool, they can be stored in a plastic box in the fridge or freezer. Once they are required, spread the cooked side with filling, roll them up, and place them snugly together in a warmed, ovenproof dish. Smother them with a tasty sauce (see pp. 157–9), then bake them in a moderate oven, 350°F (180°C) Gas Mark 4, for 20 minutes.

FILLINGS

Chopped mushrooms and onions, fried and in a thick sauce make a succulent filling. 'Cream style' sweetcorn is also very good, either alone, or with prawns, tinned salmon, or tuna, stirred into it. Or try a filling of 'Rissol-Nut' Cream as in the following recipe.

MAIN COURSES WITHOUT FISH 107

'Rissol-Nut' Cream

Very useful as a filling in savoury pancakes, or with pasta.

1 medium onion
2 tablespoons oil
2 tablespoons flour
$\frac{1}{2}$ pint (300ml) vegetable stock or water
2 tablespoons Granose 'Rissol-nut'

Peel the onion and cut it into chunks. Fry it gently in the oil until it is soft. Stir in the flour, and continue to cook until it foams, then add the stock or water and cook on, still stirring, until the sauce thickens.

Stir in the Rissol-nut and cook gently for 5 minutes, then taste, and add salt as necessary. Serve hot.

Hungry-Time Pancakes

This is an adaptation of an old Highland recipe dating back to a time when obesity was unimaginable among crofters. It makes a very filling snack, or can be served with vegetables to make a main meal. Do not eat very frequently!

1 small onion
$\frac{1}{2}$ large carrot
3 egg-whites
1 tablespoon soya sauce
1 tablespoon oatmeal
2 tablespoons vegetable oil

Peel the onion and slice thinly, and grate the carrot. (It is easier to grate half of a large carrot, than a whole small one.) Put the egg-whites into a bowl with the soya sauce and the oatmeal. Stir this mixture.

Warm the oil in a medium-sized non-stick frying pan, and cook the onion and carrot very gently until they are soft. Add the egg mixture to the pan, and fry until lightly browned.

108   MAIN COURSES WITHOUT FISH

Toss or turn and fry the other side. Serve at once.

Yorkshire Pudding, or Popovers

Traditionally, Yorkshire pudding, or popovers (which are little individual Yorkshire puddings cooked in small metal dishes or patty pans), are served with gravy, *before* the roast meat. We, however, normally serve them with 'gravy' of our own kind, and a selection of vegetables, as a main course in their own right, the protein content being the egg-white as well as whatever protein is in the vegetables and wholemeal flour.

> 2 oz (50 g) wholemeal flour
> Pinch of cooking salt
> 2 egg-whites
> ¼ pint (125 ml) water
> 1 tablespoon vegetable oil

Sift the flour and salt into a bowl, adding the bran which is left in the sieve. Make a 'well' in the centre of the flour, and pour in the egg-whites and a little of the water. Using a wooden spoon, stir in the flour, gradually adding more water as necessary to make a smooth batter, and beat lightly. Stand the batter aside for at least 30 minutes before using it.

Heat the oven to hot, 425°F (220°C) Gas Mark 7. Put the oil into a shallow baking tin, or divide it between small dishes, and put into the oven until the oil is smoking hot. Remove, and pour the batter into the tin or tins, return to the oven, and bake for 50 minutes. Serve at once.

For the 'gravy', see pages 157–8.

Potato Latkes

A tasty and substantial Jewish dish which we eat as a main course, with a salad or green vegetable.

> ½ lb (200 g) potatoes

MAIN COURSES WITHOUT FISH   109

$\frac{1}{2}$ tablespoon finely chopped onion
1 tablespoon flour
2 egg-whites
Cooking salt
Vegetable oil

Peel the potatoes and grate into a mixing bowl. Add the onion and the flour, and stir in the lightly beaten egg-whites and the salt. This mixture should be soft enough to drop from a spoon. If it is too dry and stiff, add another egg-white.

Heat some oil in a pan, and drop in spoonfuls of the mixture. Fry until brown on both sides, and serve straight away.

Pizza

$\frac{1}{4}$ oz (7 g) fresh yeast, or $\frac{1}{2}$ teaspoon dried yeast
$\frac{1}{2}$ teaspoon honey
5 tablespoons tepid water
4 oz (100 g) wholemeal plain flour
$\frac{1}{4}$ teaspoon cooking salt
1 egg-white
2 tablespoons vegetable oil
2 tablespoons flour
1 teaspoon curry powder
$\frac{1}{4}$ pint (125 ml) vegetable or fish stock
Suitable fish, shellfish and/or vegetables to decorate

Mix the yeast with the honey and a little of the water. (If using dried yeast, leave the mixture in a warm place for about 10 minutes, until it is frothy. Fresh yeast can be used at once.)

Mix the wholemeal flour and salt in a bowl. When the yeast is ready, add it and the egg-white to the remaining water, and stir into the flour mix in the bowl. Knead to a smooth dough, and continue kneading for a further 5 minutes. (This is quite hard work, and can best be done with a dough-hook on an electric mixer, to save painful hands.)

MAIN COURSES WITHOUT FISH

Press the dough out into a disc on a floured, raised-edge baking sheet, spreading it out as thin as possible in the space. Cover with a clean teatowel, and leave in a warm place for 15 minutes while you prepare a very hot oven, 475°F (240°C) Gas Mark 9, and make the topping sauce.

To do this, heat the oil and stir in the flour and curry powder. Cook gently until it froths and then add the stock, and continue stirring until the sauce is very thick and smooth.

When the pizza dough is ready, spread the sauce evenly over it and decorate with pieces of fish and vegetable. Cook for 10–15 minutes and serve at once.

Mushroom Soufflé

> ½ lb (200 g) mushrooms
> 3 tablespoons vegetable oil
> 2 tablespoons flour
> ½ pint (250 ml) vegetable stock or water
> Cooking salt
> 4 egg-whites

Chop or slice the mushrooms, and fry them in the oil. Add the flour, and when it froths, add the stock or water. Bring to the boil, stirring all the time, and cook until it thickens. Taste, and add salt as required. Allow this sauce to cool a little.

Whisk the egg-whites very stiffly, then fold them into the mushroom-sauce mixture. Pour into a greased soufflé dish (2 pint/1 litre size) or an ovenproof dish, and bake in a moderately hot oven, 400°F (200°C) Gas Mark 6, for 45 minutes. Serve at once.

Note: We like to have baked potatoes with this dish, to give 'body' to the meal. They should be scrubbed, pricked, and put on the top shelf of the oven before you begin to make the soufflé, as they require about an hour (according to their

MAIN COURSES WITHOUT FISH 111

size) to cook through. Eat the potato skins—they are most nutritious as well as tasty.

Macaroni in Onion Sauce

This is a useful supper dish, being a reasonable substitute for macaroni cheese, which it tastes remarkably like, but it is a bit short on protein.

> 4 tablespoons macaroni (wholewheat or white)
> Cooking salt
> 1 large onion
> 1 tablespoon flaked almonds (optional, but adds valuable protein)
> 1 tablespoon vegetable oil
> 2 tablespoons flour

Cook the macaroni in plenty of boiling, salted water, until soft. This will take about 15 minutes, but do read the packet, as different makes do vary.

Peel and chop the onion, and fry it and the almonds, if used, very gently in the oil, until the onion is soft, and the macaroni almost ready. Lift the onions and nuts out of the oil, and keep them warm.

Sprinkle the flour into the oil and cook until it froths, then add some of the water from the macaroni pan, and cook to a thick sauce. Stir in the onion and nut mixture, and simmer gently.

When the macaroni is done, drain it in a sieve, and stir it into the sauce. Serve.

DRIED PULSES

Dried beans, peas and lentils are an excellent source of protein, and anyone on Dr Dong's Diet will do well to make good use of them. Pulses can form the basis of several good main course dishes. I have only given three actual recipes

112 **MAIN COURSES WITHOUT FISH**

here, because such a variety of others can be found in existing cookery books (see pp. 181–2).

Unfortunately the protein is what is called 'incomplete', and cannot be utilized by the body unless eaten along with other foods, such as grains. Thus the traditional 'baked beans on toast' is a grand dish from the nutritional standpoint *if* the toast is made with wholemeal bread. Unfortunately for us, most commercial baked beans are tinned in tomato sauce, so Dong Dieters cannot make use of them. Pinto beans are normally tinned without harmful additives, and are almost as nice served on wholemeal toast.

Dried pulses should be carefully examined, and any stones or any beans which are not nice looking should be discarded. Then put them into a sieve and wash well under running water. This done, place the beans in a large container (they swell), and cover with plenty of water, to soak for about 10 hours. If tiny bubbles begin to appear, you have soaked them unnecessarily long.

It is essential to discard the soaking water, and to rinse the beans very well before cooking. This is because beans contain trisaccharides, which are indigestible to humans, and tend to cause flatulence. Fortunately, the trisaccharides are water-soluble, so most of the flatulent effects can be prevented by discarding the soaking water and washing.

Blackeye beans (sometimes called blackeye peas), split peas and lentils can all be cooked without soaking.

If you possess a pressure-cooker, then you should use it to cook peas or beans, as they take a very long time at room pressure. If not using a pressure-cooker, bring a large pan of water to a fast boil, and then drop the beans in gradually, so that boiling does not stop. When all the beans are in, reduce heat and simmer for 30 minutes, then discard the water, add fresh water to cover the beans again, bring to the boil and simmer until the beans are soft. The time varies with the type of bean, but may take several hours. Do not allow the pan to boil dry!

Kidney beans contain poisons and should never be eaten

MAIN COURSES WITHOUT FISH 113

raw or half-cooked. They must be boiled vigorously (not simmered) for at least 10 minutes to destroy the poisons. If you are going to cook them in a slow cooker, boil them properly first.

If using a pressure-cooker, you must proceed as the manufacturer advises. Some pressure-cookers work at 10 lb pressure, and some 15 lb. The higher pressure takes only half the time.

Below are suitable pressure-cooking times for most of the common types of bean available in Britain.

PULSE	NEEDS SOAKING	MINS @ 10 lb	MINS @ 15 lb
Adzuki (red) beans	Soak	25/30	10/15
Black beans	Soak	25/30	10/15
Blackeye beans (peas)	——	15	6/10
Brown beans	Soak	25/30	10/15
Butter (Lima) beans	Soak	20	10
Chick peas (garbanzos)	Soak	25/30	10/15
Garbanzos (chick peas)	Soak	25/30	10/15
Great Northern beans	Soak	25/30	10/15
Haricot beans	Soak	20	10
Kidney beans	Soak	25/30	10/15
Lentils	——	15	6/10
Lima (butter) beans	Soak	20	10
Navy (pea) beans	Soak	20	10
Pea (navy) beans	Soak	20	10
Peas—split	——	15	6/10
Peas—whole, dried	Soak	25/30	10/15
Pink beans	Soak	20	10
Pinto beans	Soak	20	10
Red (adzuki) beans	Soak	25/30	10/15
Soup (whole dried) peas	Soak	25/30	10/15
Soya beans	Soak	50/60	25/30
Split peas	——	15	6/10
Whole dried (soup) peas	Soak	25/30	10/15

114 MAIN COURSES WITHOUT FISH

After cooking, it is better to allow the pressure to reduce slowly, as fast reduction tends to burst the beans.

Foogath of Beans

The protein in this dish comes from beans and onion. It should be eaten with another dish containing protein.

$\frac{1}{2}$lb (200g) haricot or butter (Lima) beans
2 teaspoons yeast extract
4 tablespoons vegetable oil
1 onion
1 teaspoon ground ginger
1 tablespoon desiccated coconut

Soak the beans, drain and cook with yeast extract and water to cover.

Heat the oil, and fry the peeled and sliced onion gently until tender, add the beans, ginger, and coconut. Heat through, and serve very hot.

Blackeye Beans with Marjoram

$\frac{3}{4}$ pint (375ml) blackeye beans (peas)
$1\frac{1}{2}$ pints (850ml) vegetable stock or water
1 bayleaf
$\frac{1}{2}$ cup chopped onion
3 tablespoons long-grain rice (white or brown)
1 teaspoon cooking salt
1 teaspoon dried marjoram
3 tablespoons vegetable oil

Put all the ingredients into the pressure-cooker. Cook at pressure for 15 minutes (10lb) or 8 minutes (15lb).

When the pressure has reduced, remove the lid, warm through again in the open pan, and serve with a green vegetable.

MAIN COURSES WITHOUT FISH 115

Lentil Pilau

$\frac{1}{2}$ pint (250 ml) lentils
$\frac{3}{4}$ pint (375 ml) bulgar (parboiled cracked wheat)
$\frac{1}{2}$ teaspoon cooking salt
3 pints (1·7 litres) vegetable stock or water
1 teaspoon yeast extract
2 tablespoons vegetable oil
1 medium onion

Rinse the lentils and put them into a pressure-cooker or a generous saucepan with the bulgar, salt, stock or water, yeast extract, and 1 tablespoon of the oil, and cook until the lentils are soft.

Meanwhile peel the onion and slice it thinly. Fry it in the remaining oil until it is soft and golden brown, turning occasionally. If using a pressure cooker for the lentils, reduce pressure quickly.

Serve the lentil and bulgar mixture with half of the onions on each helping. A green vegetable, or a salad, goes very well with this dish.

Vegetable Dishes

ARTICHOKES

There are two kinds of artichoke: globe and Jerusalem. Globe artichokes are a sort of flower, growing at the top of a tall plant. Jerusalem artichokes are a root vegetable, rather like long, thin, lumpy potatoes. The flavour of the two kinds is somewhat similar.

Globe artichokes should be as fresh as possible. A particularly nice variety have in-curved leaves, so that the head resembles a chrysanthemum. Cut the stem close to the head, and remove the lowest ring of the petal-like leaves, as these will be tough and unpleasant to eat. Wash the heads very thoroughly, and soak them in cold water for half an hour; then drain, upside down.

Boil in salted water for 20–40 minutes, until the leaves can be pulled off easily. Again drain upside down, then serve hot, one to each person, with an egg-cup of olive oil to dip each leaf in. (Non-arthritics will doubtless prefer melted butter!)

To eat the artichoke, pull off each leaf with your fingers, and dip the soft part into the oil, then suck it, scraping the fleshy bit off with your teeth. Discard the tough upper part of the leaf (which is most of it), and pull off the next, and so on, until all the leaves are gone. Once the final, inner 'witch's hat' of leaves has been removed, the 'choke' will be exposed as a flower-like disc of thread-like, in-pointing bristles. It is well named, and quite inedible (so beware, as you approach it). Cut this away with a knife, to leave the fleshy base and butt of the stem—the most delicious and

VEGETABLE DISHES

succulent part of the whole thing, and your reward for all the work of eating the rest of it and successfully avoiding the 'choke'.

These 'artichoke hearts' can sometimes be bought tinned without additives, but the fresh vegetable is much nicer.

Do not discard the water in which you have boiled *globe* artichokes. It makes a pleasantly flavoured stock containing many of the vitamins and minerals from the heads, and can be used in making soups and sauces, or even in cooking other vegetables.

The flesh of *Jerusalem artichokes* is white, but tends to discolour after peeling. Scrub them well, and peel them (a fiddly job), then place at once in cold water. For Dong Dieters, one cannot add lemon juice or vinegar to the water, so some slight discoloration is inevitable. Add a little salt, and boil for about 30 minutes, until soft.

Do not keep the cooking water from Jerusalem artichokes, because its use as stock in soups, sauces, or whatever, will cause the most dreadful flatulence!

ASPARAGUS

Fresh asparagus should be used as soon after it is picked as possible, as it loses flavour. It is an expensive vegetable, so don't buy it unless it looks really fresh and perky. You will require 16–24 spears for 2 people.

Wash the spears well, and scrape the stems downwards with a sharp knife. Cut the longer ones so that they are all the same length, and tie in a tight bundle with string. Stand them in a saucepan, a tall one, preferably, and add water and a little salt to about half-way up the stems, then boil for 15–30 minutes, until the asparagus above the water becomes tender. Avoid over-cooking though, or the heads will go mushy. The lower ends of the stems should still be crisp.

Lift the whole bundle carefully into a serving dish, then cut and remove the string. Serve hot, with an egg-cup of

VEGETABLE DISHES

olive oil for each person (or melted butter, of course, for those who can take it!), so that the head of each spear can be 'dunked' before being sucked. Avoid trying to eat too far down the stem.

Tinned and frozen asparagus are often tender throughout, and can therefore be completely consumed, but here, as opposed to the fresh kind, a knife and fork are required, as the stems are not firm enough to hold in the fingers. The advantage is that tinned or frozen asparagus can therefore be used like a normal green vegetable with a main course.

The water in which asparagus has been cooked makes a rich vegetable stock, full of useful vitamins and minerals, and is grand for soups and sauces.

AUBERGINES (EGGPLANTS)

Buy these with care, as they deteriorate quickly after picking, and bruise easily. They should look smooth, firm, and free from patches. Inspect the end close to the stem, where deterioration tends to set in first.

Cut away the stem and its leaves, and wash the 'fruit' carefully. Aubergines are usually baked, grilled, or fried.

Baked Aubergine

> 1–2 aubergines
> Cooking salt
> Fresh breadcrumbs
> Vegetable oil

Wash or peel the aubergines, and cut into slices about $\frac{1}{2}$in (1 cm) thick. Place these in an ovenproof dish, sprinkle with salt, and cover with a good layer of fresh breadcrumbs tossed in a little vegetable oil. Cook in a moderately hot oven, 400°F (200°C) Gas Mark 6, for about 15 minutes.

VEGETABLE DISHES 119

Baked Stuffed Aubergine

    1 large aubergine
    Cooking salt
    1 large onion
    Vegetable oil
    Browned breadcrumbs, or Weetabix crumbs

When you have removed the stem and its leaves from the aubergine, boil the whole 'fruit' in a large pan of salted water for 5 minutes. Meanwhile, peel and chop the onion, and fry it in a little oil until it is soft and golden.

Cut the aubergine in half, and scoop out the flesh. If the seeds are large, discard them. Chop the flesh and mix it with the onions, filling the shells with this mixture. Sprinkle the tops with some browned breadcrumbs (or Weetabix crumbs), and bake in a hot oven, 450°F (230°C) Gas Mark 8, until the top is nicely browned.

Fried Aubergine

Peel the aubergine, and cut the flesh into thin slices. Dip in lightly beaten egg-white, then in browned breadcrumbs (or Weetabix crumbs), and fry quickly in deep or shallow fat. Serve hot.

Grilled Aubergine

Wash or peel the aubergine, and cut into thin slices. Dip these in vegetable oil to which a little salt has been added and grill for about 3 minutes on each side.

BROAD BEANS

Very young broad beans can be eaten pods and all as a salad.

To cook broad beans, first shell them, and then boil in salted water until they are soft—about 20 minutes for young

120   VEGETABLE DISHES

beans and maybe 30 minutes for older ones. They can be served alone, or in a parsley sauce (p. 157).

Discard the water used to cook the beans; it may cause flatulence if used as stock, though the pods can be boiled in water to make a benign and tasty vegetable stock which is perfectly all right.

FRENCH AND RUNNER BEANS

Both French and runner beans are usually eaten pods and all, though when runner beans are very large and old, they can be shelled and cooked like broad beans.

Very young beans can be eaten raw, as a salad. They should be washed, topped-and-tailed, and served as soon after picking as is possible.

Small French or runner beans can be cooked whole, after topping-and-tailing. Large ones should also have any tough 'strings' down the sides removed, and then should be cut into 1in (2·5cm) lengths, or else sliced diagonally. Cook in boiling salted water, until tender.

Both French and runner beans can be bought tinned or frozen.

French Beans with Onion

    ½lb (200g) French beans
    Cooking salt
    1 medium onion
    1 tablespoon vegetable oil
    ½ teaspoon chopped fresh mint

Wash the beans and trim them, slice if they are large. Cook in boiling salted water, for about 15 minutes until tender, then drain and keep warm.

Peel and chop the onion; warm the oil in a small pan, and fry the onion gently until it is tender but not brown. Pour off

VEGETABLE DISHES   121

as much of the oil as possible, and add the mint. Heat, stirring, for 1 minute. Pour this over the beans, and serve.

Green Beans in Mushroom Sauce

½lb (200g) French or runner beans
Cooking salt
¼lb (100g) button mushrooms
2 tablespoons vegetable oil
2 tablespoons flour
½pt (300ml) vegetable stock or water

Wash, trim and, if necessary, slice the beans, and cook them in boiling salted water for about 15 minutes, until tender. Drain them and place them in a warm serving dish, and keep hot.

While the beans are cooking, wash the mushrooms, and slice thinly. Fry them in the oil until they are tender, remove them from the pan, and keep hot.

Stir the flour into the remaining oil, and mix well. Cook for about 2 minutes without browning, then add the stock or water, and bring to the boil, stirring continuously. Cook until the sauce is thickened, then remove from the heat, stir in the mushrooms, and pour the whole sauce over the beans. Serve hot.

Oven-Cooked Green Beans

½lb (200g) fresh or frozen French or runner beans
Cooking salt
Vegetable oil

If using fresh beans, cook them for 5 minutes in boiling water and drain. If using frozen beans, pour boiling water over them to thaw them.

Oil a large sheet of foil, place the beans on it, and sprinkle with salt. Fold the foil loosely round the beans, and place this parcel on a baking sheet. Bake in a moderately hot oven,

VEGETABLE DISHES

400°F (200°C) Gas Mark 6, for 35 minutes. Serve hot.

DRIED BEANS

For recipes for cooking dried beans, see pages 112–14.

BEAN-SPROUTS

China's favourite vegetable, eaten cooked or raw. Packed full of really concentrated goodness, bean-sprouts contain all the vitamins and minerals required to grow a full-blown plant, and are thus an almost miraculous source of food. Cook them in a little oil, and eat sprinkled with soya sauce, or enjoy them as a crisp salad, or a crunchy sandwich filling at lunchtime.

To grow your own sprouts, put a small handful of mung or adzuki beans into a glass jar, and fasten a piece of muslin over the neck of the jar with an elastic band. Rinse the beans twice a day by pouring water in through the muslin, and tipping it out again. In a few days you will have plenty of fresh sprouts, and as soon as the roots are at least as long as the beans, the whole lot can be eaten.

Some other seeds, such as wheat and alfalfa, can be sprouted in the same way; but buy seeds packaged specially for sprouting—those sold for other purposes are often treated with heat or chemicals, and rendered unsuitable.

BEETROOT

When buying raw beetroot, be careful that the skin has not been damaged, or they will bleed when being cooked. It is difficult to buy cooked beetroot which has not had an acid, such as vinegar, added to the cooking water, or put on the beetroot later. I therefore find it safer to boil my own.

VEGETABLE DISHES

Scrub the beetroot carefully, without breaking the skin. Do not cut out blemishes at this stage. Boil in plenty of salted water. Small beetroots take about an hour to cook; larger ones up to 2 hours. When they are done, the skin is easily removed by rubbing at it, and any blemishes can now be cut away.

Sliced, or diced, they are very good when stirred into a sauce (p. 157). Grated raw beetroot can be served as a salad, and adds colour and an interestingly different flavour to a mixed salad. Sliced cooked beetroot is delicious cold.

BROCCOLI

Both purple sprouting broccoli and calabrese are usually sold as 'broccoli'. In either case, they should be washed very thoroughly, and cooked in fast boiling water for about 15–20 minutes.

Frozen 'broccoli spears' (actually calabrese), should be cooked as suggested on the packet. If you like, a little onion can be chopped, and fried in olive oil with a handful of flaked almonds and a pinch of salt. This can then be used to dress the broccoli.

Perennial broccoli, sometimes known as 'white' broccoli, has flowerets like cauliflower, and should be divided into sprigs and cooked in boiling salted water for 20–30 minutes. It can be served with or without a white sauce (see p. 157), or raw in salads.

BRUSSELS SPROUTS

Small tight sprouts are the best, but take a long time to prepare. Larger tight sprouts are much quicker, and almost as good. Very open ones are almost impossible to clean well, and should therefore be avoided.

Sprouts should be washed, and any damaged or discol-

VEGETABLE DISHES

oured leaves cut away. Cut a cross in the end of the stem, to help it to cook as quickly as the leaves, and boil in salted water for 15–20 minutes.

Brussels sprouts and chestnuts mix together beautifully to form a traditional vegetable dish. For this take 2 oz (50 g) of chestnuts to every 4 oz (100 g) of sprouts. Boil the chestnuts in water for 10 minutes, then drain and peel. Put the peeled chestnuts in a saucepan with enough water to cover them, bring to the boil, and simmer for about 40 minutes, until they are soft. (A little sugar may be added to the water, but this is a matter of taste.) Be sure not to let the pan boil dry.

Meanwhile cook the sprouts in the usual way. When both are ready, drain and mix them together, and serve.

Sprouts can also be used as a salad, well washed, and cut in quarters.

CABBAGE

Many people abroad make jokes about the English eating 'stewed cabbage'. I don't blame them! Cabbage should never be over-cooked, as this destroys much of its nutritional value as well as spoiling its flavour, wasting fuel *and* making the kitchen smell horrible! It is also bad to add bicarbonate of soda to any vegetable (as some folk do) 'to keep the colour'— this too destroys much of the goodness. The colour will not be lost if you cook the cabbage *quickly*, in only a little boiling water with a dash of salt in it. People often prefer green vegetables to be slightly crisp, *'al dente'* as the Italians put it.

Wash the plant well, shred it up, and boil in a little salted water with a lid on the pan, for between 10 and 20 minutes at the most, testing with a skewer.

Spring cabbage (spring greens or *pamphrey)* is a superb vegetable, and is available when there is very little other choice in the shops. Bright and tasty, it cooks quickly, and is very nutritious.

Drumhead, or *white cabbage*, is an astonishingly heavy

VEGETABLE DISHES 125

plant, as one discovers when buying it by weight. It can be boiled as above, or shredded and used raw in salads. Or you can stuff the leaves, as on page 83.

Savoy cabbage (I have heard this called 'bubbly cabbage' because of the appearance of the leaves) is a nicely flavoured vegetable. Cook it in the same manner as drumhead. A little shredded raw savoy looks and tastes well in a salad.

Red cabbage is normally used in sauerkraut and other dishes containing vinegar, all of which are thus unsuitable for arthritic people. I was therefore surprised when I bought one, desparate for any fresh vegetable, and cooked it as if it was a drumhead cabbage, to find it was deliciously 'different'. Since then, it has been one of our favourite vegetables.

CHINESE CABBAGE (CHINESE LEAVES)

If you are unfamiliar with this vegetable, you may think it looks like a cross between celery and lettuce. It has some of the properties of both, and can be eaten cooked or raw. An excellent winter vegetable. We usually eat the heart raw, like celery, and cook the outer leaves. Again, wash this vegetable thoroughly before using it.

Boiled Chinese Cabbage

The green leaves can be separated from the white leaf-stalks or ribs, and the two parts served separately. The green leaves should be boiled for only 10 minutes, in a little salted water, whereas the leaf-stalks will need rather longer, and should be served in a white sauce (p. 157).

Baked Chinese Cabbage

$\frac{1}{2}$ small Chinese cabbage
Cooking salt

126 VEGETABLE DISHES

Water
1 medium onion
1 tablespoon oil
2 tablespoons flour
Nutmeg
Parsley to garnish

Cut up the cabbage, and cook it in a little boiling salted water, until tender.

Meanwhile, peel and chop the onion finely, and fry it gently in the oil until it is soft. Add the flour, and cook, stirring, until it froths. The cabbage should now be cooked. Pour off $\frac{1}{2}$ pint (250 ml) of the cabbage water, topping up with extra water if necessary to make up the quantity. Add this to the flour mixture. Bring to the boil and cook, stirring all the time, until the sauce has thickened.

Fold the drained cabbage into the sauce, and put the whole thing into an ovenproof dish. Sprinkle the top with grated nutmeg, and bake in a moderate oven, 350°F (180°C) Gas Mark 4, for about 30 minutes. Garnish with parsley, and serve hot.

Stuffed Chinese Cabbage

1 egg (washed)
6 large outer leaves of Chinese cabbage
   (without blemishes)
$\frac{1}{2}$ small onion
3 oz (75 g) mushrooms
2 tablespoons cooked rice
1 tablespoon vegetable oil
Vegetable stock or water

Put the egg into plenty of water in a large saucepan, and boil for 10 minutes. During this time, dip the leaves into the boiling water for one minute each, and drain. When the egg is done, pour the boiling water away, cover the egg with cold water, and crack the shell. Remove the shell as soon as the

VEGETABLE DISHES 127

egg is cool enough to handle, then cut the egg in half and discard the yolk.

Peel and chop the onion; chop the egg-white into smallish bits; wash and slice the mushrooms; and then mix them all together with the rice and oil.

Place spoonfuls of this mixture on to each cabbage leaf, roll them up tidily, and place cosily side by side in an oiled oven-proof dish. Cover with vegetable stock or water, and bake in a moderate oven, 350°F (180°C) Gas Mark 4, for 20–30 minutes.

Serve hot, with fish.

CALABRESE

See Broccoli.

CAPSICUMS

See Peppers.

CARROTS

Carrots are a most versatile vegetable. Young new carrots can be scrubbed and eaten raw, or boiled whole. Older carrots should be scraped or peeled, and sliced or chunked and boiled, or else grated and eaten raw. If you possess a 'juicer', do try carrot juice—it is delicious.

Vichy Carrots

$\frac{1}{2}$ lb (200 g) carrots
$1\frac{1}{2}$ tablespoons vegetable oil
1 teaspoon sugar
Pinch of cooking salt
1 heaped teaspoon chopped parsley

128　　　　　**VEGETABLE DISHES**

Scrape or peel the carrots and cut into slices. Put them into a saucepan with the oil, the sugar, and the salt, and heat them, stirring continuously, until they are tender. This will take from 20–30 minutes, depending on the age of the carrots and the thickness of the slices.

Stir in the parsley and pour the carrots and oil into a serving dish. Serve hot.

Glazed New Carrots

> $\frac{1}{2}$ lb (200 g) new carrots
> 2 tablespoons vegetable oil
> 2 teaspoons sugar
> Pinch of salt
> Vegetable stock or water
> Chopped parsley to garnish

Scrub and trim the carrots, scraping them if necessary.

Warm the oil in a saucepan, and add the carrots, sugar and salt, and enough stock or water almost to cover the carrots. Cook very gently, without a lid on the pan, shaking occasionally, until the carrots are soft. Remove them and keep them warm while boiling the water in the pan rapidly, to reduce it to a thick glaze. Return the carrots, and stir gently in the glaze, over the heat, for a few minutes. When the carrots are well coated with glaze, serve them sprinkled with parsley. A most attractive dish.

CAULIFLOWER

If including cauliflower in a salad, raw, it should first be divided into flowerets.

It can be cooked whole or sprigged in boiling salted water, and is traditionally served in a thick white sauce. A large whole cauliflower may take as long as 40 minutes to cook, so when trimming it, remove a cone-shaped piece from the cut

VEGETABLE DISHES 129

end of the stem, to help it cook quickly. If divided into sprigs, it should cook in about 15–20 minutes.

Cauliflower Crunch

> ½ small cauliflower
> 1 tablespoon vegetable oil
> 2 tablespoons flour
> ½ pint (300 ml) vegetable stock or water
> Fresh brown breadcrumbs
> Vegetable oil

Wash and divide the cauliflower into sprigs. There should be enough to make 2 helpings. Boil it in plenty of salted water, until tender.

Warm the oil in a medium-sized saucepan, stir in the flour, and cook until it froths, then add vegetable stock or water (but *not* the cauliflower water), and cook, stirring, until it thickens.

Drain the cauliflower, and add to the sauce, discarding the water. Pour into an ovenproof dish.

Toss a good handful of fresh brown breadcrumbs in a little oil, and spread a generous layer over the cauliflower. Put the dish under a hot grill until the top is crisp. Serve hot.

CELERIAC

This vegetable is often called 'turnip-rooted celery'. The tops are very like celery, and can be used in the same way. The root is spherical and, after peeling, may be grated for use in salads, or boiled in salted water until tender. Small roots may be cooked whole, or larger ones diced. It takes rather a long time to cook; sometimes up to an hour. Serve hot, making a sauce with the cooking water, if you like.

Equal quantities of boiled potato and boiled celeriac

130   **VEGETABLE DISHES**

mashed together make an excellent accompaniment to white fish.

CELERY

The inner stems of celery are nice served raw. They should be well washed and stood in a jug or glass of water to keep them crisp and fresh. Some people like to dip them in a little salt when munching them.

Celery can also be cooked, and served in a sauce made from the cooking water (p. 157). Chop the celery into even lengths, about 1 in (2·5 cm) long. Cook in boiling salted water for ½–1 hour. If the stems are very large and coarse, pull away as many of the 'strings' as possible before cooking.

CHICORY

Some chicory can be eaten raw as a salad, but often it is too bitter. To cook it, wash the heads well, but quickly. Cut in half, and remove the core. Put into a pan of hot water, bring to the boil, and then drain to remove the most of the bitterness. Bring a little fresh water to the boil, add the chicory, and boil for about 30–35 minutes. Drain and serve, or make a white sauce (p. 157), but only use the chicory stock for this if it does not taste too bitter.

CHILLI PEPPERS

Should be avoided. See Peppers.

CHIVES

Chives are mildly flavoured onions, and can be used as a salad vegetable, or in recipes where a mild onion flavour is

VEGETABLE DISHES

preferred. Chopped chives can also be used in Egg-White Omelet (p. 58), or in Champ (pp. 143–4), to great effect.

CORN

See Sweetcorn.

CORN SALAD (LAMB'S LETTUCE)

Corn salad—a leaf vegetable—is, as its name suggests, entirely a salad crop. Wash it well, and use it like lettuce.

CRESS

Two kinds of cress are generally available: land cress and watercress.

Land cress, usually simply called 'cress', can be purchased still growing, in small plastic tubs, or can easily be grown at home on any window-ledge on a wad of tissue. The seeds are often sold along with mustard, which can be grown in just the same way. Cress is used in salads, and as a decoration. Simply cut off the roots.

Watercress is an excellent salad, and can also be cooked like spinach (p. 147) or made into a soup.

COURGETTES

These are a kind of small vegetable marrow, and usually have more flavour than big marrows. Really small courgettes are delicious boiled whole for about 20 minutes, until tender. Larger ones should be sliced and fried, as below.

VEGETABLE DISHES

Fried Courgettes

> ½lb (200g) courgettes
> 1 tablespoon vegetable oil
> Chopped parsley to garnish

Wash or peel the courgettes and cut them into ¼in (½cm) thick slices. Warm the oil in a small frying pan, and fry the courgette slices, turning occasionally, until they are tender and golden brown on both sides. This will take about 15 minutes. Serve hot, sprinkled with chopped parsley.

CUCUMBER

Cucumber has a bad reputation as a 'repetitive' vegetable, but this is partly because many people eat it raw, *peeled*. If the skin is eaten with the flesh, it does not 'repeat' nearly as much. Thinly sliced raw cucumber makes a lovely salad dish.

Cucumbers can also be cooked. Peel a 6in (15cm) length, and either dice it, or cut it into 4 pieces. Cook in a little oil for about 10–15 minutes, in a covered pan, and serve with a white sauce (p. 157).

EGGPLANT

See Aubergines.

ENDIVE

This is a salad vegetable, normally treated like lettuce.

FENNEL

This vegetable has feathery leaves which taste of liquorice,

VEGETABLE DISHES
133

and stems which look a bit like fat, dumpy versions of celery. The leaves can be finely chopped and used to flavour a sauce (p. 157) to serve with fish.

When cooking the stems, it is important to remove all the green leafy bits, as otherwise the whole vegetable will taste strongly of liquorice. The fennel can be cooked whole, or cut up into short lengths like asparagus. Boil in a little salted water until tender; about 20 minutes for cut fennel, and about an hour for whole heads. If you have a pressure-cooker, this can be used to cook whole fennel heads, to shorten the time. You will need either one large head, or a small one for each person. Serve hot, with a sauce if you like.

GARLIC

This is usually bought as a bulb, rather like an onion. The leaves can also be used as a flavouring, and indeed the leaves of wild garlic (ramsons) have a subtly different flavour, which is most pleasant.

Garlic is extremely good for you, but a great many people do not like the taste, which tends to 'hang on the breath' (parsley is a good antidote). It is often used as a flavouring, but sparingly! Some folk like to rub a salad bowl with a cut clove of garlic before preparing the salad, and again, a small quantity of garlic can successfully be added to sauces.

HORSE-RADISH

This is a long white root, which has a very strong flavour. It should be well scrubbed, and then grated very finely, grating down the side of the root instead of across the cut end. Interesting when added to sauces, or sprinkled on to oily fish, such as mackerel or herring. Some say it 'aids digestion'.

KALE

Kale should be well washed, and shredded, then either used sparingly in a green salad, or cooked in boiling water with a little salt, until tender.

At one time the superior size and strength of the Scottish soldier was attributed to his childhood diet of 'oatmeal and kail' (Scottish spelling). Traditionally the Scots cooked their kale in a little water in a roomy pan, and poured off the water when it was almost ready, putting in a knob of butter. (We of course should use vegetable oil in place of the butter.) They then put the lid on, and continued cooking on a gentle heat, until the kale was so tender that it could be mashed, like potato. To this was added some salt, and a small handful of oatmeal.

Allow plenty of kale; it 'boils down'.

KOHL RABI

Although kohl rabi looks like a root vegetable, it is actually an enlarged stem. To prepare it, one should cut off the leaves, and peel the globes thickly. Small globes are the nicest.

Kohl rabi can be eaten raw as a salad, either cut into strips or grated. It can be boiled whole (if small), or cut into slices, or diced. It takes between 20 minutes and 1 hour, according to the size of the pieces. It can be served hot, just as it is, or in a white sauce made from the cooking liquor (p. 157), or tossed in oil with finely chopped parsley.

LEEKS

To prepare leeks, cut off the root and remove the leaves about 2 in (5 cm) above the white part. Remove the coarse outer leaves, and wash the leeks well. Washing is very diffi-

VEGETABLE DISHES   135

cult, but it is most important, as it is awful to crunch one's teeth on a mouthful of grit! It may well be necessary to cut the leek in half lengthways, to be certain of getting rid of all the soil.

Cook in a very little boiling water, making sure the pan doesn't boil dry, until the leeks are tender. Make a white sauce (p. 157). Lay the well-drained leeks in an ovenproof dish, cover with the sauce, and bake in a moderate oven, 350°F (180°C) Gas Mark 4, for about 30 minutes. Serve hot.

LETTUCE

Wash each undamaged leaf separately in plenty of cold water, shake dry, and store in a sealed bowl in the refrigerator, to keep crisp. Serve as a salad.

Lettuce can also be cooked. Wash a whole lettuce very carefully, and drain it well. Put it into a pan with a little chopped onion and enough vegetable stock or water to come about half-way up the lettuce. Add a tablespoonful of vegetable oil, and some salt if using water or unsalted stock. Bring gently to the boil, and simmer for about 30 minutes. A sauce can be made from the liquor when the lettuce has been removed, by adding a tablespoonful of cornflour dissolved in a little water, and bringing to the boil. This sauce can be poured over the lettuce, or served separately.

MAIZE

See Sweetcorn.

MARROW

See Vegetable Marrow.

136   VEGETABLE DISHES

MARSH SAMPHIRE

See Samphire.

MUSHROOMS

The cultivated mushrooms which we buy today are very handy to prepare. All you need to do is remove the root if it is there, and wash the mushrooms. If you are lucky enough to be able to pick the much tastier wild mushrooms (being careful that they are just that and not something poisonous), they must be peeled before use. Wild ones tend to be much larger, indeed when sailing off the west coast of Scotland, we once found a mushroom on one of the islands which totally filled our large frying pan, and gave all five of us a hefty piece. We cut it like a cake! Delicious!

Mushrooms can be fried in vegetable oil, or tossed in oil and grilled, or baked in a moderately hot oven, 375°F (190°C) Gas Mark 5, for about 20 minutes. Serve hot.

A little sliced raw mushroom gives a salad a pleasing flavour and different texture.

MUSTARD

See Cress.

ONIONS

These are probably used in more savoury main-course dishes than any other vegetable, but are also extremely useful in their own right.

Unblemished whole onions can be peeled, and then boiled in salted water until tender. They should be served with a white sauce made from the liquor in which they have boiled

VEGETABLE DISHES

137

(p. 157). This is nicest done with either the tiny pickling onions, or the enormous Spanish type—they're gorgeous, either way!

Onions can also be sliced and gently fried in vegetable oil, until tender, and a deep golden brown. Be generous, because people usually want a second helping, we find.

Spring onions, or *scallions*, are used mostly in salads. Some people also like chopped onion of any kind in salads, and in sandwiches too, but quite a few don't like it raw.

PARSLEY

Parsley is normally used for decoration or in sauces. It is very rich in both vitamins and essential trace minerals, so eat it as often as possible. Use it as a salad vegetable. (Jim has often found, by the way, that when offered a sandwich at a function, the parsley decorating the plate was the only thing he dared eat, since he had no idea what was in the bread!)

PARSNIPS

These white root vegetables are surprisingly sweet, and can be used either as a vegetable or flavoured with spices such as cinnamon or ginger, and used in puddings as a fruit substitute. (And you'd never know!)

Grated parsnip also makes a pleasantly different salad.

Parsnips are very good either boiled or roasted. If they are to be boiled, scrub and peel them, then cook them either whole or in slices. If whole, boil for 30–40 minutes, until tender. If sliced, they will require only about 20 minutes. Add a little salt to the water.

To roast the parsnips, scrub and peel them, and put the

VEGETABLE DISHES

whole parsnips into an ovenproof dish or roasting tin, with some vegetable oil and a very little stock or water. Sprinkle the parsnips with a little salt; cover the dish or tin with a lid, or with foil, and bake in a very moderate oven, 325°F (170°C) Gas Mark 3 (or in the bottom of a warmer oven being used to cook the main course), for about an hour, until the parsnips are tender. This method preserves more of the goodness than boiling, but of course produces none of the tasty stock.

PEAS

Although the pea season is comparatively short, it is nowadays possible to eat good peas all year round, as they come dried, tinned, bottled and frozen, as well as being sold fresh.

Tinned peas are almost always 'coloured', so beware. If you can find unadulterated ones, they are ready to eat. Just warm them up, or drain and serve as a salad.

Bottled peas are more difficult to get, and more expensive, but they are often free of 'poisons' from the arthritic point of view. They too will be ready to use.

Frozen peas are—just wonderful! Peas are at their best only briefly after being picked from their vine, so the best freezing firms get them picked, podded and frozen in an astonishingly short space of time, thus preserving their tenderness and sweetness, as well as the full flavour and nutritional value, far better than any shop-bought 'fresh' peas ever can. The only better way I know of eating peas is to stand beside the plant, pick a pod, open it, and eat the peas there and then—which Jim and I reckon as one of life's great natural luxuries. To prepare frozen peas for cooking, follow the packer's instructions, and be careful not to over-cook. A handful of frozen peas can be added to an amazing number of dishes, to add colour, flavour and interest to the meal.

Fresh peas, newly picked, are an excellent salad. To cook

VEGETABLE DISHES 139

them however, first taste one, and if it *is* tasty, boil in salted water, or vegetable stock, for 20–30 minutes, until tender. If the pea lacks flavour or is a bit mealy, add a sprig of mint to the water when boiling—it makes all the difference.

Dried peas, see pages 111–13.

Peas à la Française

1 lb (450 g) peas
2 outside leaves of lettuce
2 very small onions
1 tablespoon vegetable oil
3 tablespoons vegetable stock or water
Cooking salt to taste

Shell the peas; shred the lettuce leaves, and cut the shreds to not more than 2 in (5 cm) lengths; peel the onions. Put all the ingredients in a pan and cook for 20–30 minutes, until the peas and onions are tender. Drain and serve.

PEPPERS

Peppers are tomato-like fruits but, as we understand it, are not forbidden by Dr Dong. (He does however object strongly to arthritic people taking even tiny amounts of peppercorns (*Piper nigrum*) or the standard ground-pepper which is made from them. That's 'ordinary' pepper, in other words.)

Peppers, on the other hand, may be green, yellow, or red, and are also called capsicums or sweet peppers. We consider chilli peppers too strong for the arthritic. Paprika is another bright red spice, obtained from the dried fruit of a Hungarian capsicum, and is thus permissible on the diet.

All kinds of peppers are used in salads, and also can be stuffed with a variety of savoury mixtures, such as 'Rissol-nut' Cream (p. 107), and baked in a moderate oven, 350°F (180°C) Gas Mark 4, for 45 minutes. Unfortunately neither

140 **VEGETABLE DISHES**

Jim nor I like the flavour, so I have no experience of recipes for them. However, it should be comparatively easy to adapt your favourite recipes.

PIMENTO

See Peppers.

POTATOES

The potato is probably the most versatile vegetable, and a useful source of protein, fibre, and vitamin C. Many people eat potatoes almost automatically every day, at least once if not two or three times. We, however, have developed a feeling that too much potato may be a bad thing for the arthritic, so Jim and I eat it only about three or four times a week. The tops of the potato plant, the shoots, and any parts of the tuber which have gone greenish in colour, are in fact poisonous, not just for arthritic folk, but for everyone—a fact that is not nearly widely enough known. With these cut carefully away, however, there are many ways of cooking potatoes, and below I give twelve methods our family enjoys.

Jacket Potatoes

Scrub 2 large, good-looking potatoes of about the same size, and remove any eyes or other blemishes. Prick them well with a fork, as they may otherwise explode in the oven (and I can assure you from experience that this covers the inside of the oven with a particularly tenacious form of mashed potato). Bake at the top of a fairly hot oven, 400°F (200°C) Gas Mark 6, for $\frac{3}{4}$–$1\frac{1}{4}$ hours, until soft when gently squeezed. Even though using an oven-cloth, take care when squeezing them, as steam may spurt out of the prick holes, which can

VEGETABLE DISHES 141

cause a nasty burn if part of your hand is in the way. Serve them hot, with salt and a little olive oil if you wish. Some people consider it more elegant not to eat the skin of their baked potato, but since this is not only the most nutritious part of the tuber, but the tastiest as well, Jim and I heartily recommend it.

Boiled Potatoes

Before boiling in salted water, potatoes can be peeled, scrubbed, or if they are new potatoes, scraped. With new potatoes, the most nutritious layer is, as it were, stuck to the skin (or the skin to it, perhaps) and this will inevitably be removed if they are peeled, rather than just lightly scraped. In the south, however, potatoes are almost always peeled, but as you go north and west, this is less often the case. Again, some people eat the skin, and others don't. Anyway, boil until tender (for about 15–30 minutes, according to size, freshness, and variety). Drain, discard the liquor, and serve hot.

Chips, or French Fried Potatoes

Use 2 large, old potatoes. Peel them and cut into slices lengthwise. Cut these slices into strips so that the chips have a square section about ¼–½in (1 cm) thick. Cover with cold water for roughly half an hour before frying, to remove some of the starch (which otherwise makes them stick together), then dry them thoroughly. Put them into the chip basket, and *slowly* lower it into hot vegetable oil. To test if the oil is hot enough, drop one chip into it, and if it rises to the surface at once surrounded by bubbles, the oil is ready. Do not allow the oil to smoke, as this damages it and makes a nasty, smelly vapour in the kitchen. Fry for about 7 minutes, then drain and serve.

Variations on chips are *game chips*, more often now called *potato crisps*, and made by cutting the potatoes into very thin

142   VEGETABLE DISHES

slices across the tuber, then proceeding as for chips, but frying for only about 3 minutes. *Matchstick potatoes* are cut like ordinary chips, but very fine and not so long, and also need only about 3 minutes to cook.

Fried New Potatoes

Scrape the new potatoes and boil them for about 5 minutes in salted water, then drain and dry them, and fry in either deep or shallow oil until golden brown. If using shallow oil, turn the potatoes frequently.

Parisienne Potatoes

Very like fried new potatoes, but are made from old potatoes made into small balls with a round vegetable scoop.

Mashed Potatoes

Boil the potatoes as above, then mash them with a dash of soya milk, using a fork or a potato ricer.

Potato Croquettes

Mash the potatoes as in the previous recipe, then mix in the white of a small egg (or part of the white of a large one), a little chopped parsley, and 1 teaspoon vegetable oil. Beat all well together, then shape the mixture into rolls or balls, and dip these in beaten egg-white, then in Weetabix crumbs. Repeat this, as a good coating helps to keep the croquettes together when they are being fried. Fry in hot deep fat for 4–5 minutes, then drain carefully and serve hot.

Duchesse Potatoes

Since arthritics cannot have the traditional egg-yolk in these, this kind of potato dish will lack its usual rich colour—but

VEGETABLE DISHES 143

will be just as good to eat. Use mashed potato, and stir in an egg-white, and enough soya milk to give a stiff consistency, suitable for piping. Use a forcing bag to form rosettes of the mix on an oiled baking sheet, and bake in a hot oven, 425°F (220°C) Gas Mark 7, until they are nicely browned. Serve hot.

Sauté Potatoes

This is a handy way to use up left-over boiled potatoes. Cut them into slices about $\frac{1}{4}$ in (0·5 cm) thick, and fry these slowly in a little oil until they are brown; turn, and fry the other side. Drain well, and serve hot, lightly sprinkled with salt. For particularly luxurious sauté potatoes, fry the slices in olive oil, and toss them in chopped parsley just before serving.

Potato Scallops

This is an excellent way to use up any coating batter left after cooking the previous meal. To make such a batter, sift 3 tablespoons flour, $\frac{1}{2}$ teaspoon baking powder, and $\frac{1}{4}$ teaspoon salt, into a small bowl, and beat in cold water until it forms a creamy coating batter. Peel the potatoes (plenty, as they are very 'more-ish' like this, though too fattening to be eaten often), cut into thin slices, rinse, dry, and dip into the batter. Fry until golden brown, and eat hot with salt.

Champ

Champ is a traditional Irish dish, and was the staple food of many poorer families before the disastrous 'Potato Famine'. Champ is always a great favourite, especially with children. To make it, you need:

Potatoes
Cooking salt

144 VEGETABLE DISHES

Spinach or (frozen) peas
Soya milk
Gravy (pp. 157–8), 'Vegerine' (p. 64), or olive oil

Boil the potatoes in salted water until they are tender, and drain. Meanwhile boil the spinach or frozen peas in a little soya milk until they too are tender, then put all together in a roomy bowl, and mash them, just as you would for mashed potato. Serve very hot. At table, each person can make a small 'well' in the centre of their potato champ, and fill it with gravy, 'Vegerine', olive oil, or, if not arthritic, the traditional knob of butter. Eat with a fork. (Children—of most ages—usually have fun trying to prevent the 'well' leaking, as they work in from the edges towards the 'special', impregnated centre of the pile.)

Ragout of Potatoes

4 small, or 8 very small, potatoes
3 small onions
1 tablespoon vegetable oil
1 tablespoon flour
½ pint (300 ml) vegetable stock or water
Cooking salt to taste
Small sprig of thyme, or a pinch of dried thyme
Sprig of parsley
Small bayleaf, fresh or dried

Peel the potatoes and onions, and cut them in half unless very small. Heat the oil in a saucepan, stir in the flour, and cook, stirring, until the flour becomes a golden brown, then add the stock or water, and continue stirring until it boils and thickens. Put all the ingredients into this sauce, cover the pan, and simmer for about 45 minutes, until the potatoes are soft. Remove the bayleaf, and serve hot.

VEGETABLE DISHES

PUMPKIN

Pumpkin, or 'squash', can be cooked as a fruit, or as a vegetable. It can be treated like vegetable marrow (p. 151), but is excellent roasted in a little oil in a fairly hot oven, 400°F (200°C) Gas Mark 6, for about an hour.

RADISHES

These are a good salad vegetable, and only need to be well washed, and served very cold. They can also be sliced or turned into 'radish flowers' by cutting across from the root end, to within $\frac{1}{4}$ in (0·75 cm) of the tops in at least three directions. These are then placed in cold water for 30 minutes or more, when the 'petals' will open out. Radish flowers make a pretty decoration for other dishes, or part of an interesting hors-d'oeuvre.

Apart from the little red radishes everyone knows, it is now possible to get a variety of other kinds, such as the long white root like a fat, anaemic carrot, or the black radish. These can be sliced, or grated, and used as a salad, the flavour being quite like the familiar red radish, but pleasingly different.

(For horse-radish, see p. 133).

SALSIFY

This is a root vegetable, a bit like a thin and very white carrot. To prepare it, wash the roots and scrape them as with new potatoes. Cut into 1 inch (2·5 cm) lengths, and put at once into cold water. Since we cannot add vinegar or lemon-juice to this, the salsify may discolour a bit. Bring it to the boil and simmer for 30–40 minutes, until tender. Serve hot, or in a white sauce.

146 VEGETABLE DISHES

SAMPHIRE

Samphire can sometimes be bought fresh, and can be picked fresher still on many saltmarshes, from mid-summer until the end of September. (This is a muddy, back-breaking job, better done by several fit people at a time.) That which is covered by every tide is said to have better flavour than the samphire on higher parts of the marsh.

In late June and July the young shoots can be pinched off the roots, and these make a tangy salad, or they can be cooked. Boil them in a little water for 10 minutes, then discard the water, add a dash of oil, and continue to cook very gently, until the spears become soft. Serve hot.

By August and September the stems have developed a woody core, and the samphire can only be picked by pulling up the whole plant. Wash them well, and do not remove the roots. Place the plants head down in a saucepan of water, and boil until the heads are tender, then drain and eat at once. Samphire cooks very quickly, but if you cannot eat it straight away, leave it standing for a few minutes in the pan of hot water. To eat it, hold the root, dip the head in olive oil, then use your teeth to draw the flesh off its woody core. An unusual hors-d'oeuvre.

SEAKALE

The leaves of *wild* seakale are thick and fleshy, and virtually inedible; but the young shoots can be cooked and eaten. *Seakale beet*, sometimes known as '*Swiss chard*', is rather like spinach, and its leaves, which have white fleshy mid-ribs, can be treated the same way as spinach, cooked in boiling, slightly salted water or vegetable stock. Serve hot in a sauce made from the liquor (p. 157).

VEGETABLE DISHES 147

SHALLOTS

These are a mildly flavoured kind of onion. Cook as for
onion (pp. 136–7).

SORREL

In Britain, sorrel is usually regarded simply as a garden
weed, although it is sold occasionally. Throughout much of
Europe, however, sorrel is considered as being an important
vegetable, which can be used in salads, or cooked like.
spinach. I sometimes add a few sorrel leaves to spinach
when cooking, to alter the flavour. If picking your own, take
only the young leaves.

In France, sorrel is often chopped finely and added to a
white sauce (p. 157), to serve with fish. Rather good.

SPINACH

When buying fresh spinach, remember that although it is
very light—a pound, or half a kilo, seems an enormous
quantity—it will actually cook down into quite a reasonable
helping for two people. I find frozen spinach purée a most
useful stand-by.

When washing fresh spinach, it is necessary to change the
water several times until there is no grit left in the bottom of
the bowl. Pick over the spinach, and remove any damaged
leaves, weeds, or roots, then put the wet leaves into a
saucepan with one or two tablespoons of water, and heat it
gently until the spinach is soft, which only takes about 10–15
minutes. Drain well, and chop very finely indeed.

Creamed Spinach

1 lb (500 g) fresh spinach, or a small pack of frozen
  spinach purée

VEGETABLE DISHES

1 tablespoon water
1 tablespoon vegetable oil
2 tablespoons flour
Pinch of cooking salt
Pinch of nutmeg

If using fresh spinach, wash it very well, in several changes of water. If using frozen purée, it helps if it can be removed from the freezer in advance, so that it has thawed by the time it is required.

Put the water into a saucepan, and add either the wet leaves or the purée (either as a solid block or thawed into a sloppy mush). Heat very gently, till the leaves are soft or the frozen block has thawed, or the purée has warmed. Whole leaves should be chopped, using two knives in the saucepan (unless it's a non-stick one!).

Heat the oil in a clean saucepan; add the flour and cook, stirring, until it foams. Add the spinach to this, along with the water in which it has been cooked. Heat gently, stirring, for about 2–3 minutes, until the whole mass has become thick and creamy. Season with salt and grated nutmeg, and serve hot.

A poached egg-white (p. 58) added to this dish turns it into an excellent snack or supper dish.

SPRING CABBAGE, OR SPRING GREENS

See Cabbage.

SPROUTS

See Brussels Sprouts.

VEGETABLE DISHES 149

SQUASH

See Pumpkin.

SWEDES

These large, yellow-fleshed Swedish turnips must be peeled very deeply, as the tough skin is rather thick. The flesh can then be cut into chunks and boiled in salted water or vegetable stock until tender, which will take about 30 minutes, depending on the size of the pieces. The cooked swede can be served as it is, or (specially good) mashed with a little oil. It can also be served roasted, like pumpkin (p. 145).

SWEETCORN

Whole corncobs are at their best when they are a pale golden yellow, not a rich deep gold, as they become mealy and tasteless when over-ripe. If you can grow your own, you can open the outer leaves to see if the cob is ready, but if it isn't, close them again carefully, to prevent the wild birds from discovering the treasure! Whole cobs can also be bought, frozen or tinned. We find the tinned ones are usually more tender and tasty than frozen ones.

To cook whole fresh cobs, strip away the leaves and the 'silk'. Cut off the stem close to the body of the cob, and boil the cobs in unsalted water (salt will only make the corn tough), for 15–20 minutes. To serve, push a short skewer or cornskewer into each end of the cob. At table, roll your cob in olive oil (butter for non-arthritics), then remove the kernels from the cob with your teeth. Quite acceptable in polite society, but Jim says it's no job for a man with a beard! Two cobs each makes a reasonable supper dish.

Sweetcorn kernels, already removed from the cobs, can be bought frozen or tinned, and can be added to many dishes to

150 VEGETABLE DISHES

give colour and texture, or served as a vegetable or on toast as a snack. Fresh kernels should be cooked in a very little water for 10 minutes; frozen ones as directed on the packet. Tinned ones only require to be heated through.

SWEET PEPPERS

See Peppers.

SWEET POTATOES

These are becoming more widely available in Britain, and can be cooked in almost any way suitable for ordinary potatoes. So far, I have simply boiled them, so can only offer this recipe:

Soak in cold water for 10 minutes, then scrub them, being careful not to break the skin. Cook in boiling salted water until they can easily be pierced with a fork, then drain and peel them quickly (a finger-burning job), and dry the flesh in the oven, or under the grill, for a few minutes. Serve very hot. You will need 1 or 2 sweet potatoes, according to size, for 2 people. Very tasty indeed!

SWISS CHARD

See Seakale.

TURNIPS

These should be peeled thickly, as the skin is tough. If they are small, they can be cooked whole; larger ones should be diced. Boil in salted water or vegetable stock until tender— about 20–30 minutes, according to size and age. Serve hot.

VEGETABLE DISHES 151

VEGETABLE MARROW

A most useful vegetable for anyone on this diet, as it can be used to make an extremely good fruit substitute!

Peel the marrow, remove the seeds, and cut the flesh into chunks. Boil these with some sugar and a little ground ginger or cinnamon, until they are translucent and tender.

Marrow can also be used as a vegetable, either by boiling in salted water or vegetable stock, or by roasting, like pumpkin (p. 145).

See also Marrow and Ginger Preserve (pp. 64–5), and Cinnamon Crumble (p. 161).

VEGETABLE SPAGHETTI

A 'new' vegetable to Britain, and one I have not yet tried, but I understand that the best method of dealing with it is to boil it whole, and then cut it in half and scoop out the spaghetti-like flesh with a fork, and eat it sprinkled with soya sauce. Being large, a large pan is needed to cope with it.

WATERCRESS

See Cress.

YAMS

Yams are another of the vegetables becoming more widely available in Britain. They should be washed, peeled, rolled in flour, and then roasted in a moderately hot oven, 400°F (200°C) Gas Mark 6, until tender. They make an interesting change!

Salad Dishes

With the exception of uncooked potato and kidney bean (poisonous), almost any vegetable can be eaten raw as a salad.

Leafy vegetables may be served as whole leaves (lettuce, cress) or shredded (cabbage, sprouts), and root vegetables can be presented whole, though more usually are grated or very thinly sliced (carrots, beetroot).

Other vegetables again may be whole (peas), sliced (cucumber), sprigged (cauliflower), and so on. The main thing is that as you will not be cooking the vegetables to tenderize them, they should be presented at table in easily eaten pieces.

Cooking sterilizes food, so *raw food must be very carefully washed*. Cooking also destroys some of the nutritious properties of vegetables, and if you have arthritis, you want to derive all the good you can from your food, so *eat lots of raw salad*. It is very important to your body's defences when it is trying to fight off a degenerative disease. Give it all the help you can.

The secret of producing a really nice salad is that the flavours, textures and colours should complement each other. We use a lot of simple dishes, such as a plate of plain, thinly-sliced cucumber (with skin), a bowl of grated carrot, a bowl of lettuce leaves, etc., but we have a number of 'made-up' salad favourites as well.

Carrot and Cucumber

> 1 medium carrot
> 1 in (2·5 cm) length of cucumber

SALAD DISHES 153

1 tablespoon undiluted soya milk
1 teaspoon granulated or demerara sugar

Wash, peel and grate the carrot. Wash, peel and dice the cucumber. Mix these together and dress with the soya milk and sugar.

Note: Vegetable marrow can be substituted for cucumber.

Green Leaf

The exact choice of leaf is of course optional.

Small leaves from the centre of a lettuce
Few sprigs of parsley
6 small sorrel leaves
2 leaves of cabbage or Chinese cabbage, whole or shredded cress and/or watercress
2 leaves from spring onions, finely chopped (optional)
1–2 spinach leaves, shredded
A little of the feathery leaves of fennel, finely chopped
1 tablespoon Special Salad Cream (p. 158)
1 tablespoon undiluted soya milk

Wash all the leaves very well, shake them dry, and mix together in a bowl. The finely chopped fennel leaf can be mixed in, or added to the dressing. Make a dressing using the salad cream and soya milk, beaten well together, or else serve the salad undressed, and hand round a bowl of the Special Salad Cream with it.

Beetroot and Sweetcorn

Good handful of grated raw beetroot
2 tablespoons sweetcorn kernels (fresh, frozen or tinned)
1 tablespoon undiluted soya milk
1 teaspoon granulated or demerara sugar

Mix everything together very well.

154 SALAD DISHES

Beetroot and Watercress

Just the same as Beetroot and Sweetcorn, but using watercress leaves instead of sweetcorn kernels.

Cauliflower and Flaked Almonds

4 oz (100 g) cauliflower flowerets
2 oz (50 g) flaked almonds
1 tablespoon Special Salad Cream (p. 158)

Divide the cauliflower into tiny flowerets, and mix everything together.

Cauliflower and Carrot

4 oz (100 g) cauliflower flowerets
1 medium carrot
1 tablespoon Special Salad Cream (p. 158)

Wash the vegetables well, and divide the cauliflower into tiny flowerets. Mix all ingredients together in a bowl.

Celery and Carrot

4 sticks of celery
1 medium carrot
1 tablespoon undiluted soya milk
1 teaspoon sugar

Cut the celery across into ½ in (1 cm) strips. Grate the carrot. Mix all ingredients together.

Celeriac and Pea

1 medium celeriac
Handful of peas
1 tablespoon Special Salad Cream (p. 158)

SALAD DISHES 155

Grate the celeriac on a coarse grater, and mix everything together well.

Cabbage Salad

This is akin to coleslaw. Shred several large cabbage leaves, removing any tough ribs, and add several other vegetables of contrasting colours, flavours, and textures, like grated carrot, grated beetroot, peas, sweetcorn, diced cucumber, etc. Mix together with some Special Salad Cream (p. 158).

Cucumber Salad

$\frac{1}{4}$ cucumber
1 teaspoon chopped mixed herbs (mint, parsley, sage, etc.)
1 tablespoon undiluted soya milk
1 teaspoon sugar

Dice the cucumber, and mix everything together well.

Almond, Pea and Sweetcorn

2 heaped tablespoons peas (fresh or frozen)
2 heaped tablespoons sweetcorn (fresh or frozen)
2 heaped tablespoons flaked almonds
1 heaped tablespoon Special Salad Cream (p. 158)

Pod the peas, and remove kernels from corncobs (or thaw frozen peas or sweetcorn at room temperature). Mix all together.

Spinach and Nut

4 oz (100 g) spinach
2 oz (50 g) grated nuts (any kind)
2 tablespoons Special Salad Cream (p. 158)

156 SALAD DISHES

Wash the spinach very carefully in at least five changes of water, to be sure all soil is removed. Remove from the water, and drain well. Spread it out on a worktop, and blot the leaves with a towel, to dry it. Shred the spinach, and mix it with the nuts and the dressing.

Swede Salad

4 oz (100 g) swede
1 heaped tablespoon peanut butter (smooth or crunchy)
Water
2 teaspoons demerara or granulated sugar

Grate the swede. Make a dressing by beating the peanut butter together with some water to form a thick cream, and stir in the swede and sugar.

Note: Kohl rabi may be used instead of swede.

Sauces

Basic White Sauce

> 1 tablespoon vegetable oil
> 2 tablespoons flour
> $\frac{1}{4}$–$\frac{1}{2}$ pint (125–300 ml) water or vegetable stock

Warm the oil, stir in the flour and cook until it froths, then add the liquid, hot or cold. Bring to the boil, stirring, and continue boiling until it thickens. If you beat the sauce vigorously at this stage, it will become 'polished' (extra smooth and shiny). You can do this with a hand-held electric mixer, but don't worry if you cannot manage this sort of refinement to begin with! When you have been truly on this diet for a while, you probably will be able to, and well-polished sauces are something to look forward to.

There are many things which can be done to this basic sauce to produce a wide variety of flavours. Chopped onion and/or mushrooms can be fried in the oil before the flour is added. Chopped herbs, such as parsley, fennel or sorrel, can be added to the finished sauce, and dried herbs can either be added, or have their flavour extracted from them by boiling in the stock or water before it is used to make the sauce.

'Gravy', and Brown Onion Sauce

> 1 tablespoon vegetable oil
> 2 tablespoons flour
> $\frac{1}{2}$ pint (250 ml) vegetable stock or water
> 1 heaped teaspoon yeast extract

Warm the oil, stir in the flour and cook till it froths, then add the stock or water. Continue to cook, stirring, until hot. Add the yeast extract, and cook until the sauce is well thickened.

If preferred, cook some finely chopped onion in the oil, to make a Brown Onion Sauce, rather than plain 'gravy'—it adds protein to the meal.

Special Salad Cream

My daughter Rona suggested that I should make a mayonnaise substitute, using mustard to emulsify the oil and give flavour and colour. The result is quite remarkable.

> 1 egg-white
> 1 tablespoon water
> ½ teaspoon dry mustard
> ½ teaspoon sugar
> ½ teaspoon cooking salt
> Vegetable oil (about 1 small teacupful)

Put the egg-white and water into a liquidizer-goblet or mixer-bowl and add the mustard, sugar, and salt. Whisk together and dribble in the vegetable oil while doing so, until the mixture begins to thicken. Continue whisking, now adding the oil *very* gradually, until the thickness you like has been achieved. Store in a refrigerator. If it separates, stir it.

Basic Sweet Sauce

> 3 tablespoons cornflour
> 1 tablespoon water
> ½ pint (300 ml) sweet liquid (e.g. sugar, golden syrup or
>   honey dissolved in water)

Dissolve the cornflour in the water, in a cup or small bowl. Bring the sweet liquid to the boil, and add the cornflour.

SAUCES 159

Cook, stirring, until the sauce thickens and becomes transparent.

Syrup Sauce

    1 tablespoon vegetable oil
    2 tablespoons flour
    ½ pint (250 ml) water
    1 large tablespoon golden syrup

Warm the oil in a saucepan, and add the flour. Cook, stirring, until it foams, then stir in the water, and bring to the boil. Cook for 3 minutes, then stir in the syrup. Serve hot with puddings.

Sweet Cream

    1 egg-white
    2 tablespoons sugar

Whip the egg-white until it is so stiff that it holds its shape. Whip in the sugar, adding more, if you want.

This cream can be stored in a fridge overnight.

Puddings and Sweets

As you will see, we have not given many 'sweet' recipes, partly because the absence of fruit and milk from the diet makes such things difficult, but really because, strictly, one should not eat such things at all if arthritic, owing to the disastrous effects of carrying any excess weight, however little. Just *once in a while* though, it does no real harm to indulge in a 'safe' treat of this kind.

Syrup Tart

When Jim first tried the diet, this was the only pudding I could think of!

> 4 oz (100 g) shortcrust pastry (p. 166)
> 5–6 tablespoons golden syrup
> 2 oz (50 g) fresh breadcrumbs

Roll out the pastry and line a 7 in (17 cm) pie plate. Pour the syrup on to the tart, letting it spread over the centre, but not on to the border, which can be decorated how you like. Sprinkle the breadcrumbs on the syrup, and bake in a hot oven, 425°F (220°C) Gas Mark 7, for about 20 minutes, until the pastry border is nicely browned. Serve hot or cold.

Syrup Sponge Pudding

> 2 large tablespoons golden syrup
> 4 oz (100 g) self-raising flour
> 1 teaspoon baking powder
> ½ teaspoon cooking salt

PUDDINGS AND SWEETS 161

4 oz (100 g) castor sugar
6 tablespoons vegetable oil
2 egg-whites
2 tablespoons water

Put the syrup in a 1 pint (500 ml) ovenproof dish. Sieve together the flour, baking powder, and salt, then add the sugar. Make a 'well' in the centre of this, and pour in the oil, egg-whites, and water. Beat the mixture very thoroughly, and pour it over the syrup in the dish. Bake in the middle of a moderate oven, 350°F (180°C) Gas Mark 4, for 40 minutes. Serve hot.

Cinnamon Crumble

Vegetable marrow, about 4 in (10 cm) cut from a marrow
1 tablespoon soft brown sugar
1 teaspoon cinnamon
2 oz (50 g) Trex
4 oz (100 g) flour
2 oz (50 g) granulated sugar

Cut some vegetable marrow into 1 in (2·5 cm) dice. Stew these gently in a little water, until they begin to soften, then add the soft brown sugar and cinnamon, and continue cooking for a further 5 minutes. Remove the 'fruit', placing it in an ovenproof dish, and pour the juice over it. There should be just enough to come half-way up the 'fruit'. If there is too much, first reduce the quantity by boiling.

Rub the Trex into the flour, and stir in the granulated sugar. Sprinkle the mixture over the marrow, and bake in a moderate oven, 350°F (180°C) Gas Mark 4, for 30–40 minutes. If the oven is hotter, bake on a lower shelf, beneath some other dish. (Be economical!)

162 PUDDINGS AND SWEETS

'Fruit'

The 'fruit' used in the Cinnamon Crumble (p. 161) is made from vegetable marrow stewed together with sugar and cinnamon. It can be most useful for other puddings, like a 'Fruit Pie', for instance. It tastes really good—not a bit like marrow, oddly enough.

Chestnut Meringue Pudding

Sweetened or unsweetened chestnut purée can be used for this dish, but as the meringue itself is very sweet, I prefer the unsweetened variety of purée.

> 1 small tin of chestnut purée
> 2 egg-whites
> 4 oz (100 g) soft brown sugar, sieved

Spread the chestnut purée in a shallow dish (ovenproof). Whip the egg-whites until they are stiff and hold their shape. Add half the sugar, and whip for 2–3 minutes. Fold in the rest of the sugar. Spread or pipe the meringue over the purée, and bake in a moderate oven, 350°F (180°C) Gas Mark 4, for 10 minutes. Serve warm or cold.

Angel Cream

This superb dish, which is extremely luxurious, being made solely from egg-whites, ground almond and sugar, is one of the many marvellous recipes appearing in the two books written by Dr Dong and Jane Banks. It appears on page 214 of *New Hope For the Arthritic*, and on page 137 of *The Arthritic's Cookbook*. I feel it would be unfair of us to steal their thunder by quoting it here, but most heartily recommend it for a real treat.

Meringues

    2 whites from large eggs
    4 oz (100 g) castor sugar

Whip the egg-whites until they are very stiff and hold their shape. Sprinkle on 1 oz (25 g) of the sugar, and whip again for 2–3 minutes. This really thorough whipping makes all the difference to the quality of the finished meringues.

Fold in the rest of the sugar very gently. Line a baking sheet or two with lightly oiled greaseproof or non-stick silicone paper, and drop on to it spoonfuls of the mixture (keeping them well apart), or pipe the meringue on in fancy shapes.

Meringues are best dried out, rather than baked. This can be done in a very cool oven, 250°F (130°C) Gas Mark ½, or even in a warm airing cupboard. It will take as much as and maybe more than 1½ hours. When they are done they are 'set', and can be lifted off the paper easily, without collapsing.

To make a meringue base, use the same mixture, but draw a circle (round a plate) on to the paper before lining the baking sheet with it, and smooth the meringue mixture into a disc on it, before cooking.

Individual meringue nests, made from this mixture, can be filled with our 'Fruit' recipe (p. 162), or with 'eggs' made from a stiff paste of ground almonds, egg-white and a *little* sugar.

The same meringue mixture can be used as a topping for puddings, in which case cook in a moderate oven, 350°F (180°C) Gas Mark 4, for only 10 minutes, so that the outside is set and tinted golden brown, while the inside is still soft.

Special Christmas 'Mincemeat'

    1 parsnip, peeled, chopped, and boiled
    1 carrot, grated and boiled

164 PUDDINGS AND SWEETS

A few flaked almonds
A little preserved ginger, cut in small pieces
1 tablespoon soft brown sugar
Pinch of powdered nutmeg
Pinch of powdered mace
Pinch of powdered cinnamon
A little desiccated coconut

Mix all these ingredients in a small pan with some stock from the vegetables, and boil for 20 minutes. A little rum or whisky can be added. Use to make Mince Tarts at Christmastime—they taste incredibly like the 'real thing'!

Mince Tarts

Shortcrust or flaky pastry (pp. 166–7)
Special Christmas 'Mincemeat' (see above)
Beaten egg-white

Roll the pastry to about $\frac{1}{8}$ in (3–4 mm) thick. Use a suitable biscuit-cutter to cut rounds to line some $2\frac{1}{2}$ in (6 cm) patty tins, and a slightly smaller cutter to cut lids for them. Line the oiled tins with the larger rounds. Fill with 'mincemeat', dampen the edges, and place the lids in position. Press together to seal. Make a neat cut in the top of each pie to allow the steam to escape (I use scissors for this), and brush the tops with beaten egg-white, to glaze.

Bake towards the top of a hot oven, 425°F (220°C) Gas Mark 7, for 15–20 minutes, until they are nicely browned. Cool on a wire rack. They can be served cold, but are delicious warm. Dust with icing sugar for extra effect, and reheat in the oven before serving.

Avocado Demerara

1 avocado pear
Demerara sugar

PUDDINGS AND SWEETS 165

Cut the avocado in half, remove the stone, then carefully scoop out the flesh without damaging the skins, and cut into small dice. Put the diced flesh into a small bowl, and mix it with some demerara sugar. Return the mixture to the 2 halves of the skin, and sprinkle with a little more sugar.

Cook under a hot grill for about 5 minutes before serving.

Creamed Avocado

1 egg-white
2 tablespoons sugar
1 avocado pear

Beat the egg-white until it is very stiff, then beat in the sugar, to form a sweet cream.

Cut the avocado in half lengthways, and remove the stone. Scoop out the flesh into a bowl, without damaging the skins, and mash it until it is creamy, then stir in some of the cream (which allows you to use the rest for something else—it keeps well in a fridge). Return the mixture to the avocado skins, and cook under a hot grill for about 5 minutes before serving, hot.

Pastry, Cakes, Buns and Biscuits

PASTRY

The basic rule for making pastry is to use a pure vegetable fat, such as Trex, in place of butter, margarine, or lard.

Shortcrust Pastry

> 4oz (100g) plain flour
> Pinch of cooking salt
> 2oz (50g) Trex
> 3½–4 tablespoons cold water

Mix together the flour and salt, and cut the Trex into it with a knife. When the Trex is in small pieces, rub it in for 2–3 minutes. The mixture will then look like fine breadcrumbs, and if you shake the bowl, the lumps which come to the top will be crumbly. If there are still any lumps of fat visible, I'm afraid you have not rubbed for long enough!

The water should be added gradually, stirring the mixture all the time with a knife. When it begins to stick together, you have enough water (the exact quantity depending partly on the quality of the flour, partly on the humidity of the day, and partly on the amount of flour, so I can only give a rough guide). Collect the mixture together, and knead lightly for a few moments, to make a smooth dough. Pastry is better if it is allowed to 'rest' for about 15 minutes, before being rolled out.

Roll out the dough on a floured worktop, being very careful not to stretch it, as it will shrink in cooking if it has been stretched at this stage. Shortcrust pastry is normally

PASTRY, CAKES, BUNS AND BISCUITS 167

rolled to about ⅛in (3mm) thick, and cooked in a hot oven, 425°F (220°C) Gas Mark 7.

Shortcrust Pastry made with Oil

> 2½ tablespoons vegetable oil
> 1 tablespoon cold water
> 4oz (100g) flour
> Pinch of cooking salt

Beat the oil and water well together until they form an emulsion, then beat in the flour and salt, until a dough is formed. Knead this, rest it, and roll it as for Shortcrust Pastry above. It is a rather greasier crust than normal shortcrust, so is more suitable for savoury dishes than for sweet ones.

Flaky Pastry

> 4oz (100g) flour
> Pinch of cooking salt
> 3oz (75g) Trex
> 3½–4 tablespoons cold water

Sift together the flour and salt. Crush the Trex with a knife until it is creamy and soft, then divide it into 4 equal portions, and rub one of these into the flour. Add the water (as for Shortcrust Pastry), knead, and roll into an oblong on a floured worktop.

Divide the oblong into 3 equal sections, by marking it lightly with a knife. Using one portion of Trex dot it evenly over one end section and the middle one, then fold the other end over the middle one. Fold the fat-dotted end over this, and seal the edges by pressing them with the rolling pin. Turn the pastry so that it is at right-angles to its last position, and repeat the rolling and fat-dotting twice, thus using up all the Trex. Now wrap the pastry in a Trex paper wrapping, or in foil, and rest it in a cool place (the fridge), for at least 30 minutes, before continuing.

168 PASTRY, CAKES, BUNS AND BISCUITS

Pastry is best cooked in a hot oven, 425°F (220°C) Gas Mark 7. Flaky pastry can be glazed by brushing it with beaten egg-white, but be careful that the egg does not run down the sides, as this would seal them, and so prevent the pastry from rising.

Choux Pastry

This is usually used for cream buns and chocolate éclairs. It can, however, be used for a savoury, by filling the shells with prawns or shrimps in a thick sauce (for instance); or, to make a substitute for the real thing, a sweet cream can be made with stiffly beaten egg-white and some sugar. And do remember that waist-line!

> 8 tablespoons water
> ¼ teaspoon cooking salt
> 2 oz (50 g) flour
> 4 tablespoons vegetable oil
> 3 unbeaten egg-whites

Bring the water to the boil, and add the salt, flour and vegetable oil all at once, then stir vigorously until the mixture leaves the sides of the pan in a compact ball. Allow it to cool slightly.

If you have an electric mixer, transfer the lump of dough to the mixer-bowl at this stage. Gradually add the egg-whites while beating, and continue beating for 10 minutes, by which time it should all be smooth and glossy-looking.

Drop dessertspoonfuls of the mixture on to 2 ungreased baking sheets, keeping each spoonful at least 2 in (5 cm) apart. Bake in a moderately hot oven, 400°F (200°C) Gas Mark 6, for 30–40 minutes, until the choux puffs are light and dry inside.

PASTRY, CAKES, BUNS AND BISCUITS 169

CAKES AND BUNS

Victoria Sandwich Cake

> 5 oz (125 g) self-raising flour and
> 1 heaped teaspoon baking powder, or
> 5 oz (125 g) plain flour and
> 3 level teaspoons baking powder
> 1 teaspoon cooking salt
> 4½ oz (115 g) castor sugar
> 7 tablespoons vegetable oil
> 3 egg-whites
> 2½ tablespoons water

Sift the flour, salt, and baking powder into a bowl, and add the sugar. Make a 'well' in the centre, and pour in the oil, egg-whites, and water, beating them with a wooden spoon. Continue to beat for at least 2 minutes. If using an electric mixer, put all the ingredients into the mixer-bowl as above, and beat for at least 2 minutes.

Brush two 7-in (17-cm) sandwich tins with vegetable oil, and line the bases with circles of greaseproof or non-stick silicone paper. Divide the mixture evenly between these two tins, and bake in the centre of a moderate oven, 350°F (180°C) Gas Mark 4, for 35–40 minutes. When cooked, the cakes will spring back if pressed gently with a finger. Allow to cool in the tins for a few minutes before turning out to cool properly on a wire rack. Spread with Trex 'Cream' Filling (like butter cream, but made with pure vegetable fat—(see p. 170), and sandwich the two cakes together.

Coffee Sandwich Cake

This variation of the above recipe is simply made by dissolving a tablespoon of instant coffee in the water, before adding it to the mixture.

170   PASTRY, CAKES, BUNS AND BISCUITS

Fairy Cakes

Make the same mixture as the Victoria Sandwich (p. 169) but divide it up between patty tins or small paper cases. Bake near the top of a moderately hot oven, 400°F (200°C) Gas Mark 6, for 15–20 minutes.

Trex 'Cream' Filling

> 2 oz (50 g) Trex
> 4 oz (100 g) castor, icing, or soft brown sugar
> 1 tablespoon warm water
> Flavouring (coffee, vanilla, rum, etc.)

Beat the Trex to a smooth cream, and gradually beat in the sugar and water. Flavouring, such as a few drops of rum or some instant coffee, can be added to the water. This cream is really very good, for filling or decoration.

Walnut Cake

> 7 oz (175 g) self-raising flour
> 1 oz (25 g) cornflour
> 3 oz (75 g) chopped walnuts
> 2 teaspoons baking powder
> Pinch of cooking salt
> 5 oz (125 g) soft brown sugar
> 7 tablespoons vegetable oil
> 5 egg-whites
> A few whole shelled walnuts to decorate

Mix together the flour, cornflour, chopped walnuts, baking powder and salt, and stir in the sugar. In another bowl, mix the oil and egg-whites, then beat this very thoroughly into the dry ingredients, using a mixer if you have one. Put this mixture into a 7-in (17-cm) cake tin, which has first been oiled and lined (or use a non-stick tin).

Decorate the top of the cake with a few whole walnuts, and bake in the centre of a moderate oven, 350°F (180°C) Gas

PASTRY, CAKES, BUNS AND BISCUITS 171

Mark 4, for 1–1½ hours. To test if the cake is done, push a warm skewer into the middle of it, and withdraw it at once. If it comes out clean, the cake is ready. Allow to cool in the tin for a little while before turning it out to cool properly on a wire rack.

Rock Buns

> 3 oz (75 g) self-raising flour, or 3 oz plain flour and 1 teaspoon baking powder
> Pinch of cooking salt
> 1 oz (25 g) ground rice
> ¼ teaspoon mixed spice
> 1½ oz (40 g) demerara sugar
> 1 egg-white
> 2 tablespoons water
> 2 tablespoons vegetable oil
> 1–1½ oz (25–40 g) crystallized ginger

Sift the flour, baking powder (if used), salt, ground rice, and spice, into a bowl, and add the sugar. Mix well.

Beat together the egg-white, water and oil. Stir this into the dry ingredients, to make a 'dropping' consistency.

Cut the ginger into small pieces, and stir them into the mixture. Place heaped dessertspoonfuls well apart on greased baking trays, as they will spread while cooking.

Bake in a hot oven, 425°F (220°C) Gas Mark 7, for 10–12 minutes. Cool on a wire rack.

Hot Cross Buns

This recipe makes rather a lot, but the buns freeze very well, so can be made before Holy Week, frozen in suitable batches for a day's use, and enjoyed all week.

> 4 fl oz (100 ml) boiling water
> 6 fl oz (150 ml) cold water
> 1 slightly heaped tablespoon dried yeast
> 2 tablespoons brown sugar

172 PASTRY, CAKES, BUNS AND BISCUITS

1 lb (450 g) flour (wholemeal is very good)
$\frac{1}{3}$ teaspoon cooking salt
$\frac{1}{2}$ teaspoon mixed spice
2 tablespoons vegetable oil, or 1 oz (25 g) Trex
1 egg-white

Mix the boiling and cold water in a measuring jug. Sprinkle on the yeast and sugar, and leave the jug in a warm place until the mixture has frothed up well. This will take about 10 minutes.

Meanwhile, sift the flour, salt and spice into a bowl, and rub in the Trex, or stir in the oil. Make a 'well' in the centre, and when the yeast has frothed, pour it in. Add the egg-white, and mix until a dough forms, then knead for at least 5 minutes. This is best done with an electric mixer.

Cover the bowl with a clean teatowel, and leave it to stand in a warm place (see notes about this in the bread section on p. 61) for about an hour, until it has doubled in size.

Knock back the dough, and reknead it, then divide it up into balls, about 2 in (5 cm) across. Place these on a floured baking sheet, mark with a cross, using a sharp knife to cut the surface of the dough. Cover with the teatowel again, and put back into the warm place to 'prove' for about 20 minutes.

Bake in a moderately hot oven, 400°F (200°C) Gas Mark 6, for 10–15 minutes. These buns should be glazed by brushing the tops with a mixture of beaten egg-white and brown sugar, while they are still very hot. Cool on a wire rack.

Rich Dark Gingerbread

5 oz (125 g) solid vegetable oil
5 tablespoons treacle
7 oz (175 g) wholemeal plain flour
2 rounded teaspoons ground ginger
2 egg-whites
2$\frac{1}{2}$ oz (80 g) soft brown sugar
2 tablespoons water
$\frac{1}{4}$ teaspoon bicarbonate of soda

PASTRY, CAKES, BUNS AND BISCUITS 173

Put the solid vegetable oil and the treacle into a small pan, and heat gently until the oil is melted. Meanwhile, sieve the flour and the ginger into a roomy bowl, returning the bran to the flour once this is done.

Mix together the egg-whites and sugar in a small bowl, and mix in a cup the water and bicarbonate of soda.

When the oil has all melted, pour the treacle and oil into the flour mixture; add the egg-white mixture and the water, and mix all very well together. An electric mixer helps a lot.

Line a swiss-roll tin with oiled greaseproof paper or non-stick silicone paper, and pour the mixture into it. Bake in the centre of a moderate oven, 350°F (180°C) Gas Mark 4, for 20–25 minutes. To test when it is done, press gently with a finger. If the cake springs back when the finger is removed, it is ready.

Cool on a wire rack, and cut into squares. If you want to keep it, just cool it in the tin, then wrap it in foil, and store in a cool place. It keeps very well.

Crumbly Gingerbread

This is a kind of ginger-flavoured shortbread, and can be kept for up to 3 weeks in an airtight tin.

9 oz (200 g) flour
1 teaspoon bicarbonate of soda
1 teaspoon cream of tartar
$\frac{1}{2}$ teaspoon ground ginger
4 oz (100 g) soft brown sugar
2 oz (50 g) crystallized ginger
6 tablespoons vegetable oil
1 slightly heaped tablespoon golden syrup
2 teaspoons granulated sugar

Sift the flour, bicarbonate of soda, cream of tartar, and ground ginger into a bowl, and add the soft brown sugar. Chop the crytallized ginger finely, and add it to the mixture.

174 PASTRY, CAKES, BUNS AND BISCUITS

Make a 'well' in the centre, and pour in the oil and syrup, and mix thoroughly. (An electric mixer helps no end!)

Press the mixture into a tin; sprinkle it with the granulated sugar, and bake in the centre of a very moderate oven, 325°F (170°C) Gas Mark 3, for 45–50 minutes.

Cool in the tin for 15 minutes, then cut into wedges or fingers. Turn out, and cool on a wire rack.

Ginger 'Gunge'

    6 oz (150 g) self-raising flour, or 6 oz plain flour and 2 teaspoons baking powder
    3 teaspoons ground ginger
    6 oz (150 g) rolled oats
    9 oz (225 g) soft brown sugar
    ½ pint (1250 ml) vegetable oil
    1 heaped tablespoon golden syrup

Sieve the flour, baking powder (if used) and ginger together. Stir in the oats and the sugar.

Melt the vegetable oil, add the syrup, and pour this into the dry ingredients, mixing thoroughly.

Line a baking tin, about 8 × 10 in (20 × 25 cm), with oiled greaseproof or non-stick silicone paper, and pour in the mixture. Bake in a very moderate oven, 325°F (170°C) Gas Mark 3, for about 45 minutes.

Allow to cool in the tin, and cut into fingers.

Golden Pops

This recipe is adapted from one on the Rice Krispie packet. Hard vegetable oil, such as Pura, is necessary to make these 'set'. If liquid oil or Trex is used, the result will be very sticky.

    4 tablespoons golden syrup
    ½ oz (15 g) castor sugar
    ½ oz (15 g) solid vegetable oil
    3 oz (75 g) Rice Krispies

PASTRY, CAKES, BUNS AND BISCUITS   175

Put syrup, sugar and oil into a pan and warm over a low heat, stirring occasionally until the oil is dissolved, then bring to the boil for 1 minute.

Remove from the heat. Mix the Rice Krispies into the melted ingredients, and ensure that they are all coated. Oil a 7-in (17-cm) square tin, and press the mixture down into it firmly.

Leave until cold, then cut into 16 squares.

BISCUITS

Coffee Biscuits

7 oz (175 g) plain flour
1 oz (25 g) cornflour
2 heaped tablespoons sugar
2 teaspoons dry instant coffee
2 tablespoons water
6 tablespoons vegetable oil
1 slightly heaped tablespoon golden syrup

Sieve together the flour and cornflour, and stir in the sugar. Dissolve the coffee in the water, add the oil and syrup, and mix together. Beat the liquids into the dry ingredients (an electric mixer helps), to make a stiff dough.

Roll out, and cut with a biscuit-cutter. Put the biscuits on to an oiled baking sheet, and press the remaining dough together, then cut some more. Repeat this until only a tiny piece of dough is left, and shape even that into a biscuit.

Bake in a moderate oven, 350°F (180°C) Gas Mark 4, for about 20 minutes. Cool on a wire rack. Makes about 30 biscuits.

176   PASTRY, CAKES, BUNS AND BISCUITS

Yorkshire Ginger Biscuits

>7 oz (175 g) flour
>1 oz (25 g) cornflour
>1 teaspoon ground ginger
>2 teaspoons baking powder
>½ teaspoon bicarbonate of soda
>6 oz (150 g) sugar
>4 oz (100 g) golden syrup
>6 tablespoons vegetable oil

Sift the flour, cornflour, ginger, baking powder and bicarbonate of soda into a bowl, and add the sugar.

In another bowl, mix the syrup and the oil. Pour this into the dry ingredients, and mix until a thick dough is formed. Roll this out on a floured board, and cut with a biscuit-cutter. Place the biscuits on an oiled baking sheet and bake in a moderately hot oven, 375°F (190°C) Gas Mark 5, for about 15–20 minutes, until the biscuits are golden brown. Cool on a wire rack. Makes about 30 biscuits.

Note: Alternatively, one can use cinnamon instead of ginger.

Oat and Nut Biscuits

>1 tablespoon golden syrup, black treacle, or molasses
>8 tablespoons vegetable oil
>4 oz (100 g) soft brown sugar
>3 oz (75 g) porridge oats
>2 oz (50 g) chopped nuts or flaked almonds
>4 oz (100 g) wholemeal flour
>2 teaspoons bicarbonate of soda

Melt the syrup, treacle or molasses with the oil and the sugar, over a low heat. Stir in all the remaining ingredients, and mix well. Allow to cool a little.

Roll the mixture into small balls, about 1 in (2·5 cm) across,

PASTRY, CAKES, BUNS AND BISCUITS 177

and place these well apart on oiled baking sheets. They will spread when cooking.

Bake in a cool oven, 300°F (150°C) Gas Mark 2, for about 20 minutes. Cool on a wire rack. Makes about 35 biscuits.

Oat Biscuits

    3 oz (75 g) Trex
    1 tablespoon rum
    1 slightly rounded tablespoon golden syrup
    3 oz (75 g) flour
    $\frac{1}{2}$ teaspoon bicarbonate of soda
    3 oz (75 g) demerara or soft brown sugar
    3 oz (75 g) rolled oats

Melt the Trex in a large saucepan, together with the rum and syrup.

Mix all the remaining ingredients together, and stir them into the liquid in the pan. Mix very thoroughly, and stand it aside for a few minutes.

When the mixture is cool enough to handle comfortably, roll pieces of it between the hands to form 1 in (2·5 cm) balls. These should be placed on a greased baking sheet, well spaced out as the biscuits spread when cooking.

Bake in a very moderate oven, 325°F (170°C) Gas Mark 3, for about 25–30 minutes.

Allow the biscuits to cool and set on the trays for a few minutes before attempting to lift them on to a cooling rack. Makes about 20–25 biscuits.

Almond or Coconut Biscuits

    $3\frac{1}{2}$ oz (90 g) self-raising flour
    $\frac{1}{2}$ oz (15 g) cornflour
    1 teaspoon baking powder
    4 oz (100 g) ground almonds or desiccated coconut
    4 oz (100 g) sugar

178 PASTRY, CAKES, BUNS AND BISCUITS

7 tablespoons vegetable oil
1 tablespoon golden syrup

Sift together the flour, cornflour and baking powder. Stir in the almond or coconut, and the sugar.

In another bowl, mix the oil and syrup, then stir these into the dry ingredients, mixing very well. An electric mixer helps!

Roll the mixture between the hands into small balls, about 1 in (2·5 cm) across, and put these well apart on oiled baking sheets. Bake in a moderately hot oven, 375°F (190°C) Gas Mark 5, for about 15 minutes. Cool on a wire rack. Makes about 22 biscuits.

Peanut Butter Cookies

$4\frac{1}{2}$ oz (115 g) flour
$1\frac{1}{2}$ oz (40 g) cornflour
1 teaspoon baking powder
6 oz (150 g) soft brown sugar
5 tablespoons corn oil
1 heaped tablespoon peanut butter (smooth or crunchy)
1 egg-white

Sift together the flour, cornflour, baking powder and soft brown sugar.

In a roomy bowl (a mixer-bowl if you have one) mix the corn oil, peanut butter, and egg-white, until they form a thick cream, then beat in the dry ingredients.

Roll this mixture between the hands to form small balls about 1 in (2·5 cm) across, and place them well apart on an oiled baking sheet. They spread when cooking. Bake in a moderately hot oven, 375°F (190°C) Gas Mark 5, for 10–15 minutes.

Allow to cool on the tray for only 2–3 minutes before moving them on to a wire rack. If they become cold on the baking tray, they will be too brittle, and will stick. Makes about 22 biscuits.

PASTRY, CAKES, BUNS AND BISCUITS 179

'Cheese' biscuits

These little biscuits taste so 'cheesy' that people who know about the diet have been known to enquire if Jim should really be eating them. (There's not a scrap of cheese in them!)

    1 tablespoon water
    1 teaspoon yeast extract
    3oz (75g) flour
    Cooking salt
    1oz (25g) soya flour
    1oz (25g) Trex
    Egg-white to glaze

Warm the water, and dissolve the yeast extract in it.

Sift the flour, salt and soya flour into a bowl, and rub in the Trex. Mix in the yeast extract and water, to make a stiff dough.

Roll out the dough, and cut with a small biscuit-cutter, or cut with a knife into 'straws', and brush with lightly beaten egg-white, to glaze. Bake on an oiled baking sheet, in a moderately hot oven, 375°F (190°C) Gas Mark 5, for about 15 minutes. They should then be golden brown. *If removed too early from the oven they have no flavour*.

Cool on a wire rack, and serve with drinks.

LIFE ON DR DONG'S DIET CAN BE FULL OF PLEASANT SURPRISES!

Useful Books

The Arthritic's Cookbook by Collin H. Dong and Jane Banks (Granada, 1974).
New Hope for the Arthritic by Collin H. Dong and Jane Banks (Granada, 1976).

Both of these are wonderfully helpful books, but unfortunately for British-based readers, Jane Banks's recipes are American, and many call for certain ingredients which are difficult, expensive, or even impossible to obtain in British shops, while some of our best fish and vegetables are not mentioned. This is the reason why we began to write our own book on the diet!

Diet for Life by Mary Laver and Margaret Smith (Pan, 1981).

Mary Laver wrote the article which introduced us to Dr Dong's Diet. She suffered from severe rheumatoid arthritis, and together with Margaret Smith, who is a home economist, has written a book which goes more deeply than ours into nutritional principles. Many of their excellent recipes now enrich our own diet.

The following titles are books for the general culinary reader, with no bias towards any particular diet. They therefore contain numerous unsuitable recipes for Dong Dieters, but have proved very useful to us when 'converting' from our old way of eating.

The Penguin Cookery Book by Bee Nilson (Penguin, 1971).

A very clear book, explaining how to cook, simply and extremely comprehensively. Particularly useful to anyone who has not cooked before.

182 USEFUL BOOKS

The Wholemeal Kitchen by Miriam Polunin (Heinemann and *Here's Health*, 1977

Excellent for those unaccustomed to baking with wholemeal flour.

Not Just a Load of Old Lentils by Rose Elliot (Fontana, 1972).

The best vegetarian cookery book we know.

Index

Acids, 24, 26: ascorbic, 24; fruit, 24; vinegar, 26
Adapting recipes, 51
Additives, chemical, 16, 18, 24, 40
Alcohol, 26, 27 (*see also* Beer and Wine)
Allergies, 21, 22
Almonds: biscuits, 177; in salad, 154, 155; trout with, 90
Angel cream, 162
Angler fish (monkfish) 44–5: 'scampi', 92
Animal fat, 18, 35
Arthritic, New Hope for the, 22, 66, 162, 181
Arthritic's Cookbook, The, 22, 162, 181
Artichokes, globe and Jerusalem, 116–17
Asparagus, 117–18
Aubergine (eggplant), 118–19: baked, 118; baked stuffed, 119; fried, 119; grilled, 119; pâté, 68
Avocado, 27, 46: creamed, 165; demerara, 165; with prawns, 67; supreme, 67

Balm, lemon, 34: in drinks, 55
Banks, June, 22, 181
Batter, 81
Beans: dried, 111–15; French, with onion, 120; green, in mushroom sauce, 121; green, oven-cooked, 121
Bean-sprouts, 122
Beer, 55: ginger, 55–6
Beetroot, 122–3; in salad, 153, 154; soup, 76
Biscuits, 31, 44, 48: almond or coconut, 177; 'cheese', 179; coffee, 175; oat, 177; oat and nut; 176; Yorkshire ginger 176
Bleeding, 23
Bread, 27, 31, 36, 60–3: soda, 62; yeast, 61
Breakfast, 28, 29, 30
Breakfast cereals, 30, 57
Broccoli, 123
Brown onion sauce, 157
Brussels sprouts, 123–4
Buns: hot cross, 171; rock, 171

Cabbage, 124: in salad, 155; stuffed, 83–4; (*see also* Chinese cabbage)
Cakes: coffee sandwich, 169; fairy, 170; filling for, 170; Victoria sandwich, 169; walnut, 170
Calabrese (broccoli), 127
Capsicums (peppers), 139–40
Carrots, 127–8; glazed new, 128; in salad, 152, 154; Vichy, 127
Carrot juice, 54–5, 57, 127
Catarrh, 19

INDEX

Cauliflower, 128–9: crunch, 129; in salad, 154
Celeriac, 129–30; in salad, 154
Celery, 130: in salad, 154
'Cheating', 17, 36–8
'Cheese' biscuits, 179
Chestnut, 29: meringue pudding, 162; in nut roast, 101–2
Chicken: breast, 27, 36; broth, 27; roast, 101
Chicory, 130
Children, 34
Chilli peppers, 139–40
Chinese cabbage (Chinese leaves), 125–7
Chinese restaurants, 33
Chives, 130–1
Christmas: dinner, 29; special mincemeat, 163
Cinnamon: in biscuits, 176; crumble, 161
Coconut biscuits, 177
Cod, 79, 82, 83: salt, 86
Coffee, 27, 30, 54: biscuits, 175; sandwich cake, 169
Colouring, 40
Consommé, instant, 71
Convenience foods, 14, 39–40
Corn (see sweetcorn)
Corn salad (lamb's lettuce), 131
Cortisone, 14, 23
Courgettes, 131: fried, 132
'Cream' filling, 170
Cream, sweet, 159
Cress, 131
Croutons, 77
Crumble, cinnamon, 161–2
Cucumber, 55, 132: in salad, 152, 155
Curry powder, 27

Diet for Life, 181
Dinner menus, 29

Dong, Collin H., 21–3, 181
Dr Dong's Diet, 26–8
Drinks, alcoholic, 26–7, 55
Drinks, soft, 27, 54
Drugs, use of, 14, 23

Eating out, 32–4, 35–6
Egg 'mayonnaise', 69
Eggplant (see aubergine)
Egg-whites, 27, 41, 51: fried, 59; 'mayonnaise', 69; omelet, 58; poached, 58; scrambled, 59
Endive, 132
Entertaining, 34–5
Exercising, 24–5

Fairy cakes, 170
Fat, vegetable, 47
Fennel, 132–3
Fish, 27, 31, 44–5, 79–99; in cabbage leaves, 83; casserole, 82; Chinese-style, 84; crumble, 83; foil-baked, 79; fried, 80; grilled, 80; kedgeree, 87; pasties, 81; poached, 79; smoked, 85; tinned, 42
Fish soups, 71–4
Flour, 27, 52
'Fruit', 161
Fruit acids, 24, 26, 45

Garlic, 52, 133
Ginger, 30: biscuits, Yorkshire, 176; 'gunge', 174; and marrow preserve, 64
Ginger beer, 55
Gingerbread: crumbly, 173; rich dark, 172
Golden pops, 174
Gravy, 157
Green leaf salad, 153

Haddock, 79, 82, 83, 87: bake, 86

INDEX

185

Hairy tatties, 86
Health foods, 42–4
Here's Health, 15, 182
Herring: fried, 88; stuffed, 88
Honey, 27
Hors-d'oeuvres, mixed, 66
Horse-radish, 133
Hot cross buns, 171

'Jam', 65
Juices, vegetable, 54–5, 57, 127

Kedgeree, 87
Kale, 134
Kohl rabi, 134: in salad, 156

Lamb's lettuce, 131
Laver, Mary, 16, 17, 19, 22, 181
Leeks, 134–5
Lentils, 111, 113: pilau, 115
Lettuce, 135
Lunch, 28, 29, 30

Macaroni: in onion sauce, 111
Mackerel: baked, 89; baked
    stuffed, 89; poached stuffed,
    89; stuffed, 89
Maize (*see* sweetcorn)
Margarines, 27, 47
Marrow, 151: in cinnamon
    crumble, 161; and ginger
    preserve, 64; as 'fruit', 162
Marsh samphire, 146
'Mayonnaise', egg, 69
Medicines, use of, 14, 23
Menus, 28–9
Meringue, 29, 163: and chestnut
    pudding, 162
Milk, cow's, 51
Milk, soya, 30, 42, 43, 57
'Mincemeat', Christmas, 163
Mince tarts, 29, 164
Mint, 55, 56

Monosodium glutamate, 18, 26,
    32, 33, 36, 40, 43, 45
Mushroom, 136: soufflé, 110;
    soup, cream of, 77; soup,
    with egg-whites, 74
Mussels: in vegetable sauce, 97
Mustard, 27

New Hope for the Arthritic, 26, 66,
    181
Not Just a Load of Old Lentils, 182
Nuts, 27, 47: in biscuits, 176–8;
    products, 43–4, 105, 107;
    roast, 101; in salad, 155 (*see
    also* almonds)
'Nuttolene', 44, 105

Oats: biscuits, 176–7; oaty nosh,
    57; in porridge, 57
Oils, 47–8
Onion, 136–7: sauce, brown,
    157; soup, 75

Pancakes, 105; 'hungry-time',
    107
Parsley, 137
Parsnip, 137: soup, 77
Pasta, 26, 28: pink (with
    prawns), 96
Pastry, 166–8: choux, 168; flaky,
    167; shortcrust, 166;
    shortcrust with oil, 167
Pâté, 67, 68: aubergine, 68;
    tuna, 68
Peanut butter, 30: cookies, 178
Peas: dried, 111–14; green,
    138–9; à la Française, 139; in
    salad, 154, 155
Penguin Cookery Book, The, 181
Pepper, 18, 26, 33
Peppers, 139–40
Pinto beans, 44, 113
Pizza, 109
Plaice, 79, 82, 83

INDEX

Plant milk, 30
Popovers, 108
Porridge, 57
'Postum', 29, 54
Potato, 46, 140–4: boiled, 141; champ, 143; chips, 141; croquettes, 142; duchesse, 142; fried new, 142; jacket, 140; latkes, 108; mashed, 142; parisienne, 142; sauté, 143; scallops, 143
Prawns: and avocado, 67; in dragon sauce, 94; flan, 95; and pasta, 96; soufflé, 95; and vegetables, 93
'Protose', 43, 104
'Protoveg', 43: hot-pot, 102; shepherd's pie, 103
Pudding, 160–5
Pulses, 111–15
Pumpkin, 145

Radishes, 145
Rice, 27, 46
'Rissol-Nut', 43: cream, 107
Rock buns, 171
Rum, 27, 52, 55

Salad, 152–6
Salad cream, special, 158
Salmon: cakes, 90
Salsify, 145
Salt, 27
Samphire, 146
Sandwich cake: coffee, 169; Victoria, 169
'Sandwich Spread', Granose, 68
Sauces, 157–9
Scones, 63
Seafood, 32, 45: recipes, 79–99
Seakale, 146
Seasoning, 27
Shallots, 147

Shellfish, 27, 45: recipes, 67, 93–9
Shepherd's pie, 103
Side-effects of diet, 21, 23–4
Smith, Margaret, 181
Soda water, 27, 54
Sole, 79, 82, 83
Soufflé: mushroom, 110; shrimp or prawn, 95
Soup, 71–8: beetroot, cream of, 76; fish, Doris's, 73; fish, quick, 70; fish, thick, 73; French onion, 75; mushroom, cream of, 77; mushroom, with egg-white, 74; parsnip, cream of, 77; spinach, 78; sweetcorn, cream of, 76; vegetable, 75
Spinach, 147; in champ, 143; in salad, 155; soup, 78
Sponge pudding, 160
Spring cabbage, 124
Spring greens, 124
Sprouts, 123–4
Squash, 145
Steroid drugs, 14, 23
Sugar, 27, 52
Supper, 28
Swede, 149; in salad, 156
Sweets (candy), 32, 44; (puddings), 160–5
Sweetcorn, 41, 149–50: in salad, 153, 155; soup, 76
Sweet cream, 159
Sweet potato, 150
Swiss chard, 146
Syrup, 27, 52: sauce, 159; sponge pudding, 160; tart, 160

Tarts: mince, 164; syrup, 160
Tea, 27, 28, 29, 30: varieties, 54
Textured Vegetable Protein, 27, 43, 51

INDEX

187

Tinned fish, 42
Travelling, 35–6
Trex 'Cream' filling, 170
Trout: with almonds, 90
Tuna: hot-pot, 91; pâté, 68
Turkey: breast, 27; roast, 101
Turnip, 150

'Vegerine', 30, 48, 64
Vegetables, 27, 46–7, 116–51:
 broth, 75; raw, 31; in salads,
 152–6; sauce, mussels in, 97
Vegetable fats, 48
Vegetable juice, 54–5
Vegetable marrow, 151
Vegetable oils, 27, 47, 51
Vegetable spaghetti, 151
Victoria sandwich cake, 169

Vine leaves, stuffed, 69
Vitamin C, 24
Vodka, 27, 55

Walking stick, best use of, 14,
 17, 25
Walnut cake, 170
Watercress, 131: and fish soup,
 72; in salad, 154
Weight, personal, 19, 25, 26, 32,
 35, 52, 160
Whisky, 27, 52, 55
White sauce, 157
Whiting, 79, 82, 83
Wholefood, 39
Wholemeal Kitchen, The, 181
Wine, 27, 36, 52, 55

DR DONG'S DIET

MUST NOT EAT:
Meat in any form, including broth
Dairy products (milk, cream, butter, cheese, yogurt, whey)*
Egg-yolks
Fruit of any kind, including tomatoes
Chocolate
Dry-roasted nuts (the process involves monosodium glutamate)
Pepper (definitely)
Vinegar, or any other acid
Most alcoholic beverages
Soft drinks (where they contain additives, fruit products or colouring)
Man-made 'chemical' additives (flavourings, preservatives, colourings); this applies above all to *monosodium glutamate*.

* The lecithin in margarine is acceptable, but whey is not. Beware of this.

CAN EAT:
All fish, including shellfish
All vegetables, including avocados
Parsley, onions, garlic, bayleaf, or any other of the herbs
Vegetable oils (especially safflower and corn oils) and pure vegetable fat
Margarine free from milk solids (whey) and forbidden additives
Egg-whites—only
Honey
Sugar (preferably undyed brown), syrup, etc.
Bread and other baked products containing no forbidden additives
Flour of any kind
Rice of all kinds
Soya bean products such as Textured Vegetable Protein (T.V.P.) when free from forbidden additives
Nuts and sunflower seeds
Tea and coffee, taken without milk
Plain soda water
Pure salt (beware of additives in table salt)

CAN OCCASIONALLY EAT:
A little breast of chicken or turkey, and chicken broth.
Small amount of wine in cooking
Small drink of whisky, rum, vodka, and possibly white wine (not red)
Very small pinch of spicy seasoning, such as curry powder, mustard, etc.
Pasta such as noodles, spaghetti, macaroni (when present, the amount of egg in these is small)